Occupational Medicine

Occupational Skin Disease

Guest Editor:
James R. Nethercott, MD
Department of Dermatology
University of Maryland School of Medicine
Baltimore, Maryland

Volume 9/Number 1 January–March 1994
HANLEY & BELFUS, INC. Philadelphia

STATE OF THE ART REVIEWS

Publisher: HANLEY & BELFUS, INC.
210 South 13th Street
Philadelphia, PA 19107
(215) 546-4995
Fax (215) 790-9330

OCCUPATIONAL MEDICINE: State of the Art Reviews is included in *Index Medicus, MEDLINE, BioSciences Information Service, Current Contents* and *ISI/BIOMED.*

OCCUPATIONAL MEDICINE: State of the Art Reviews **(ISSN 0885-114X)**
January–March 1994 **Volume 9, Number 1** **(ISBN 1-56053-147-9)**

OCCUPATIONAL MEDICINE: State of the Art Reviews is published quarterly by Hanley & Belfus, Inc., 210 South 13th Street, Philadelphia, Pennsylvania 19107. Second-class postage paid at Philadelphia, PA and at additional mailing offices.

POSTMASTER: Send address changes to OCCUPATIONAL MEDICINE: State of the Art Reviews, Hanley & Belfus, Inc., 210 South 13th Street, Philadelphia, PA 19107.

The 1994 subscription price is $82.00 per year U.S., $92.00 outside U.S. (add $40.00 for air mail).

Occupational Medicine: State of the Art Reviews
Vol. 9, No. 1, January–March 1994

OCCUPATIONAL SKIN DISEASE

James R. Nethercott, MD, Editor

CONTENTS

CONTRIBUTORS

Jerry E. Cooley, MD
Resident, Department of Dermatology, University of Maryland School of Medicine, Baltimore, Maryland

Chester L. Davidson, MD
Associate Clinical Professor of Medicine (Dermatology), University of Louisville, Louisville, Kentucky

Tuula Estlander, MD, PhD
Dermatologist (spec. in occupational dermatology), Department of Occupational Medicine, Institute of Occupational Health, Helsinki, Finland

Brian G. Forrester, MD, MPH
Assistant Professor, Division of Occupational and Environmental Medicine, University of Alabama at Birmingham, Birmingham, Alabama

Ronald Goldner, MD, FACP
Clinical Associate Professor, Department of Dermatology, University of Maryland School of Medicine, Baltimore; Chief, Division of Dermatology, Maryland General Hospital, Baltimore, Maryland

Daniel J. Hogan, MD
Associate Professor, Department of Dermatology and Cutaneous Surgery, University of Miami, Miami; Professor of Medicine, Public Health, and Pediatrics, University of South Florida, Tampa; Chief of Dermatology, Bay Pines VAMC, Bay Pines, Florida

D. Linn Holness, MD, MHSc
Assistant Professor, Department of Medicine, Preventive Medicine and Biostatistics, Chemical Engineering and Applied Chemistry, University of Toronto, Toronto; Chief, Department of Occupational and Environmental Health, St. Michael's Hospital, Toronto, Ontario, Canada

Riitta Jolanki, DTech (ChemEng)
Docent in Dermatotoxicology, Specialist Researcher, Department of Occupational Medicine, Institute of Occupational Health, Helsinki, Finland

Lasse Kanerva, MD, PhD
Professor and Chief, Department of Occupational Medicine, Section of Dematology, Institute of Occupational Health, Helsinki, Finland

Jack N. Moss, BSc
Formerly, Research Section Manager, Toxicology, Rohm and Haas Company, Research Division, Springhouse, Pennsylvania; Currently, retired

James R. Nethercott, MD
Professor, Department of Dermatology, University of Maryland School of Medicine, Baltimore, Maryland

J. Barrie Ross, MB, BS, RRCPC, DObstRCOG
Professor of Medicine (Dermatology), Division of Dermatology, Department of Medicine, Dalhousie University, Halifax, Nova Scotia, Canada

Kyllikki Tarvainen, MD
Dermatologist, Department of Occupational Medicine, Institute of Occupational Health, Helsinki, Finland

James S. Taylor, MD
Head, Section of Industrial Dermatology, Department of Dermatology, The Cleveland Clinic Foundation, Cleveland, Ohio

Niels K. Veien, MD, PhD
The Dermatology Clinic, Aalborg, Denmark

PUBLISHED ISSUES

(available from the publisher)

Vol 2/No 2 Apr.–June 1987	**Occupational Pulmonary Disease** Edited by Linda Rosenstock, MD, MPH University of Washington, Seattle, Washington
Vol 2/No 4 Oct.–Dec. 1987	**Workers with Multiple Chemical Sensitivities** Edited by Mark R. Cullen, MD Yale University School of Medicine, New Haven, Connecticut
Vol 3/No 1 Jan.–Mar. 1988	**Back Pain in Workers** Edited by Richard A. Deyo, MD, MPH University of Washington, Seattle, Washington
Vol 3/No 2 Apr.–June 1988	**Worker Fitness and Risk Evaluations** Edited by Jay S. Himmelstein, MD, MPH and Glenn S. Pransky, MD, MPH University of Massachusetts, Worcester, Massachusetts
Vol 3/No 3 July–Sept. 1988	**The Petroleum Industry** Edited by Neill K. Weaver, MD Washington, D.C.
Vol 3/No 4 Oct.–Dec. 1988	**Psychiatric Injury in the Workplace** Edited by Robert C. Larsen, MD, and Jean S. Felton, MD University of California, San Francisco, and Irvine, California
Vol 4/No 1 Jan.–Mar. 1989	**The Management Perspective** Edited by L. Fleming Fallon, Jr., MD, MPH, MBA, O.B. Dickerson, MD, MPH, and Paul W. Brandt-Rauf, ScD, MD, DrPH Columbia University, New York, New York
Vol 4/No 2 Apr.–June 1989	**Alcoholism and Chemical Dependency** Edited by Curtis Wright, MD, MPH The Johns Hopkins University, Baltimore, Maryland
Vol 4/No 4 Oct.–Dec. 1989	**Problem Buildings** Edited by James E. Cone, MD, MPH University of California, San Francisco, California and Michael Hodgson, MD, MPH University of Pittsburgh, Pittsburgh, Pennsylvania
Vol 5/No 1 Jan.–Mar. 1990	**Hazardous Waste Workers** Edited by Michael Gochfeld, MD, PhD, and Elissa Ann Favata, MD UMDNJ–Robert Wood Johnson Medical School Piscataway, New Jersey
Vol 5/No 2 Apr.–June 1990	**Shiftwork** Edited by Allene J. Scott, MD, MPH Navy Environmental Health Center, Norfolk, Virginia
Vol 5/No 3 July–Sept. 1990	**Medical Surveillance in the Workplace** Edited by David Rempel, MD, MPH University of California, Richmond, California
Vol 5/No 4 Oct.–Dec. 1990	**Worksite Health Promotion** Edited by Michael E. Scofield, PhD AT&T, Basking Ridge, New Jersey

1994 ISSUES

Occupational Skin Disease
Edited by James R. Nethercott, MD
University of Maryland, Baltimore, Maryland

Training in Occupational Safety and Health
Edited by Michael J. Colligan, PhD

Construction Safety and Health
Edited by Knut Ringen, DrPH, Anders Englund, MD, Laura Welch, MD, James L. Weeks, ScD, and Jane L. Seegal, MS

Tuberculosis in the Workplace
Edited by Steven Markowitz, MD
New York University School of Medicine, New York, New York

1993 ISSUES

The Mining Industry
Edited by Daniel E. Banks, MD
West Virginia University
Morgantown, West Virginia

De Novo Toxicants
Edited by Dennis J. Shusterman, MD, MPH
California EPA, Berkeley, California
and Jack E. Peterson, PhD, CIH
Alpine, California

Spirometry
Edited by Ellen A. Eisen, ScD
University of Massachusetts
Lowell, Massachusetts

Women Workers
Edited by Dana M. Headapohl, MD
St. Patrick's Hospital
Missoula, Montana

1992 ISSUES

Back School Programs
Edited by Lynne A. White
Director, Practice Management Resources
San Francisco, California

Occupational Lung Disease
Edited by William S. Beckett, MD
Yale University School of Medicine
New Haven, Connecticut
and Rebecca Bascom, MD
University of Maryland School of Medicine
Baltimore, Maryland

Unusual Occupational Disease
Edited by Dennis J. Shusterman, MD, MPH
Berkeley, California
and Paul D. Blanc, MD, MSPH
University of California, San Francisco
San Francisco, California

Ergonomics
Edited by J. Steven Moore, MD
Medical College of Wisconsin
and Arun Garg, PhD
University of Wisconsin–Milwaukee
Milwaukee, Wisconsin

1991 ISSUES

Prevention of Pulmonary Disease in the Workplace
Edited by Philip Harber, MD, MPH
University of California, Los Angeles
and John R. Balmes, MD
University of California, San Francisco

Health Hazards of Farming
Edited by D. H. Cordes, MD, MPH
and Dorothy Foster Rea, MS
University of Arizona College of Medicine
Tucson, Arizona

The Biotechnology Industry
Edited by Alan M. Ducatman, MD
and Daniel F. Liberman, PhD
Massachusetts Institute of Technology
Cambridge, Massachusetts

The Nuclear Energy Industry
Edited by Gregg S. Wilkinson, PhD
University of Texas Medical School
at Galveston
Galveston, Texas

Ordering Information:
Subscriptions for full year and single issues are available from the publisher—
Hanley & Belfus, Inc., 210 South 13th Street, Philadelphia, PA 19107.
Telephone (215) 546-7293; (800) 962-1892. Fax (215) 790-9330.

PREFACE

It is a pleasure to serve as editor of this issue of **Occupational Medicine: State of the Art Reviews** devoted to occupational skin disease. The contributing authors provide scholarly reviews of subject material germane to the field which reflect their interest and research into the subjects they have reviewed. The problem of work-related skin disease continues as one of the major challenges in occupational health. The understanding of some of the mechanisms of these diseases is improving, but standard-setting to effect primary prevention still poses a significant problem.

It is hoped that the reader will gain significant insight into a selected number of key issues in this challenging field from reading the work of the assembled experts who have contributed to this volume. Progress has been made, but much more is necessary if the needs of workers with skin disease due to work or of workers at risk for developing skin disease are to be adequately served by the professional and scientific community.

James R. Nethercott, MD
GUEST EDITOR

JAMES S. TAYLOR, MD

EVALUATION OF IMPAIRMENT DUE TO WORK-RELATED SKIN DISEASE

From the Section of Industrial Dermatology
Department of Dermatology
Cleveland Clinic Foundation
Cleveland, Ohio

BASIC DEFINITIONS

Before discussing evaluation of impairment and disability in the workplace, it is important to define terms. For the most part I use definitions from the fourth edition of *Guides to the Evaluation of Permanent Impairment*, published by the American Medical Association (AMA) in 1993.[8]

Impairment is defined as "an alteration of an individual's health status . . . a deviation from normal in a body part or organ system and its functioning . . . and the loss, loss of use, or derangement of any body part, system, of function."[8] Permanent impairment of the skin is "any anatomic or functional abnormality or loss that persists after medical treatment and rehabilitation and after a length of time sufficient to permit regeneration and other physiologic adjustments."[8] A disorder is considered to become permanent after 12 months' duration, but in fact the time frame may be longer or shorter than 1 year. The *Guides* popularized the concept that impairment is a medical issue assessed by medical means, whereas disability is a nonmedical assessment generally determined by adjudicating authorities.[8]

Disability is defined as an "alteration . . . (decrease in, or the loss or absence) . . . of the capacity of an individual to meet personal, social, or occupational demands or to meet statutory or regulatory requirements. . . [and] refers to an activity an individual cannot accomplish . . . and may be thought of as the gap between what a person can do and what the person needs or wants to do."[8] It is important to remember that an impaired person is not necessarily disabled. The classic example often cited is that of two individuals who lose the distal portion of the phalanx of the same finger. Although impairment for both persons is the same, disability is likely to be greater for the individual who is a concert pianist than for the individual who is a bank president.[8]

A handicap exists "when an impairment is associated with an obstacle to useful activity . . . that can be overcome only by compensating in some way for the effects of the impairment, [through the] use of assistive devices, such as crutches, wheelchairs, elevators, hearing aids, optical magnifiers, prostheses, or special tools or equipment. Accommodation may include modification of the environment."[8]

Definitions by Other Systems

Other definitions of impairment, disability, and handicap are provided by the World Health Organization, the Americans with Disabilities Act (ADA), the Social Security Administration, the Veterans Affairs Department, and various federal laws, to name a few.[2-4,8,11,14] Chapter 1 and the glossary of the AMA *Guides* provide succinct definitions and discussion of many of these systems, including federal employees', railroad, and maritime workers' compensation. The ADA has direct relevance to workers' compensation (see chapter 2 in this issue by Nethercott).

IMPORTANCE OF DISABILITY FROM OCCUPATIONAL SKIN DISEASE

According to statistics from the U.S. Bureau of Labor,[9,15] work-related skin disorders were the second most common cause of occupational diseases in the United States in 1992. The number of cases of skin disease (62,900 in 1992) has actually increased since 1980, although skin diseases now account for a smaller percentage of the total number of reported illnesses (14% in 1992 vs. 43% in 1980). The major reason for the apparent discrepancy is the dramatic increase in diseases associated with repeated trauma (e.g., carpal tunnel syndrome), which represented 18% of cases (approximately 25,000) in 1980, whereas in 1992 they accounted for 62% of cases (281,800). In 1984, when federal statistics were last available on time lost from work, approximately 25% of workers with occupational disease lost time from work, averaging 10–12 days each. Other statistics, outcomes, factors that affect outcome, and social consequences of occupational disability have been discussed by Nethercott.[13]

WORKERS' COMPENSATION

In essence, workers' compensation laws are no-fault statutes that hold employers responsible for the cost of occupational injury and disease claims while guaranteeing benefits to covered workers who meet the law's requirements. Although all states now recognize responsibility for occupational diseases, this area of law still has the greatest variability among the states. Evaluating physicians should become familiar with their own state workers' compensation laws, regulations, and definitions by consulting various references, such as the yearly *Analysis of Workers' Compensation Laws*,[2,5] and by contacting the medical director of the state workers' compensation system, state and local medical and occupational medical societies, or local attorneys who specialize in compensation law for both workers and companies. Some states have specific written information or manuals for physicians. The AMA *Guides*[8] are mandated, recommended, or frequently used in 40 of 53 jurisdictions (38 states and 2 territories).

In general, three types of payment may be made when a claim is approved:

1. Temporary total disability payments to compensate for lost wages;
2. Payment of medical bills; and
3. Payment for permanent partial or permanent total disability.

Temporary partial impairment occurs when the impaired person returns to work but at a lower wage. Under workers' compensation laws, disability is equivalent to economic loss, for which the affected worker is to be compensated.[2]

Most claims based on occupational skin disease involve temporary total or permanent partial disability. It is important for the examining and treating physician to know when temporary total impairment ceases. In Ohio[16] this occurs with one of the following events:

1. The patient has reached maximal medical improvement or is "medically stationary";
2. The condition has become permanent;
3. The patient has a valid job offer within his or her physical capabilities;
4. The patient states that he or she is capable of returning to work; or
5. The patient returns to work.

Athough time-loss compensation may cease, the worker is often still entitled to compensation for medical services related to the condition.

Some states allow third-party liability suits arising out of workers' compensation cases. As an example, a machinist who received workers' compensation for patch-test–proved allergic contact dermatitis to a coolant germicide also sued the manufacturer of the germicide for damages from injury.

EVALUATION OF PUTATIVE OCCUPATIONAL DERMATOSES

Dilemmas for the Physician

Medical determinations in workers' compensation involve a number of issues for the examining and treating physician:[1]

1. Patient assertions and demands concerning work-relatedness of their disease, job changes, and job modifications;
2. Social gate-keeping concerning time off from work, date for return to work ("Why can't it be on Friday?"), and determination of work-relatedness of disease;
3. Lack of adequate workplace data, such as detailed job descriptions, lists of work contactants and exposures, including material safety data sheets, and in some cases samples of workplace chemicals. This is probably the major deficiency facing the physician. A plant visit is ideal but often not practical;
4. Clinical judgment versus technology; for example, determining whether a machinist with hand eczema and negative patch tests has an occupational irritant contact dermatitis; and
5. Conceptual differences in medical versus legal concepts of causation. Absolute proof fulfilling Koch's postulates is not required in workers' compensation cases. Determination by the physician that a cause-and-

effect relation exists between a disease and a job "within a reasonable medical certainty or probability" is usually adequate. Statement of a "possible" relationship is not adequate.

Medical Evaluation

The patient history is an integral part of the evaluation. Published history forms may be used by physicians or their assistants or adapted for self-administration by patients.[6,7] An initial examination of the area of chief complaint often helps to direct the questioning. The history of the present illness should focus on the following:

1. Patient's description of the chief complaint(s);
2. Chronology, including duration and frequency of occurrence;
3. Location of the lesions at onset;
4. Spread, if any;
5. Morphology of the lesions;
6. Time away from work, including weekends, vacations, sick leave, and disability; and
7. Accidental versus usual exposure to chemicals.

Determination of the timing of the reaction also is important. Onset of symptoms within minutes or 1–2 hours points more to contact urticaria or irritation. Onset after 1–2 days or as long as 1 week suggests contact allergy, especially in first-time cases of dermatitis or in recurrent, intermittent acute dermatitis. This distinction is blurred in chronic cases. It is also important to remember that irritation, contact urticaria, and contact allergy may coexist. The interval between initial exposure and onset of occupational acne or pigmentary disturbance is usually several weeks; for tumors, several years.[10]

The course of occupational contact dermatitis is usually improvement away from work for a few days and exacerbation on reexposure, unless there is a common contactant both at home and at work. Exceptions to this rule clearly exist. Outcome studies in workers with industrial dermatitis, as reviewed by Nethercott,[13] show persistent dermatitis in one-third or more of cases. A number of potential reasons may account for prolonged occupational dermatitis. Treatment from the plant dispensary and physicians or self-purchased over-the-counter medications should be listed. A list of drug allergies and other medications should be included. The frequency and effect of systemic corticoids should be determined, especially for reports of improvement away from the job.

Work history should include:

1. A description of the job and job title(s);
2. List of work contactants;
3. Review of material safety data sheets;
4. Dates of employment, hours worked per week, shift, and dates and effects of any job or task changes;
5. Related complaints from other workers, if any;
6. Methods and frequency of cleaning the skin, including use of waterless hand cleansers and workplace solvents; and
7. Protective creams and protective clothing, especially gloves.

Direct questions about specific causes of flares and improvements also may be helpful.[6]

Past history should include:

1. A listing of previous compensation claims and skin conditions;
2. Allergies such as childhood eczema, asthma, and hay fever;
3. Overt reactions to the major contact allergens, such as metals, medicaments, cosmetics, dyes, and preservatives;
4. Past medical history;
5. Review of systems;
6. Family and social history; and
7. Hobbies and second jobs.[6]

In some instances, a review of old medical and hospitalization records is important.[8]

The physical examination should include the location, description, and distribution of the eruption as well as a listing of other important cutaneous findings.[6] A complete examination is often indicated. In contact allergy the area of most intense dermatitis usually corresponds to the site of most intense contact with the allergen. Exceptions to this rule exist, as when allergens are transferred to distant sites. Volatile airborne chemicals may cause dermatitis on exposed body areas. Contact dermatitis may be symmetrical or asymmetrical, uniform or confluent, or it may involve discrete patchy areas.

Results of diagnostic tests should be recorded, especially scrapings for microorganisms, cultures, laboratory tests, biopsies, and patch tests. Specific comments about their relevance should be included.

Diagnosis and Treatment

The diagnosis should be listed along with other significant cutaneous findings. Associated diagnoses, such as asthma or significant systemic illness, also should be recorded. I often list other major symptoms purported by the patient to be occupationally related and recommend appropriate evaluation by an occupational physician or other specialist. An assessment of the current medical status and statement of further medical plans and treatment also should be included.[8]

Causation

Determination of the cause-and-effect relation between a skin disorder and an occupation is not always clearcut. Key[10] lists five criteria to consider for the diagnosis of occupational skin diseases:

1. Appearance of the lesions;
2. Site of the eruption;
3. History;
4. Course of the disease; and
5. Diagnostic tests.

Mathias[12] has adapted these criteria for establishing occupational causation and aggravation in contact dermatitis. He proposes that a "yes" answer to four of the following seven questions is generally adequate to establish probable cause:

1. Is the clinical appearance compatible with contact dermatitis?
2. Are there workplace exposures to potential irritants or allergens?
3. Is the anatomic distribution of the eruption compatible with job exposure?

4. Is the temporal relationship beween exposure and onset consistent with contact dermatitis?
5. Have non-occupational exposures been excluded as causes?
6. Does the dermatitis improve away from work exposure to the suspected irritant or allergen? and
7. Do patch or provocation tests identify a probable cause?

Impairment Evaluation

As a prelude to impairment evaluation, the physician must determine the impact of the medical condition on life activities and whether or not the condition is stable and unlikely to change.[8] If the worker has a new or recent-onset condition that significantly precludes working on the current job, then temporary total impairment may exist, and an appropriate amount of time away from work may be warranted under most workers' compensation laws. Unduly restrictive limitations, such as avoiding all contact with a particular substance, may jeopardize a worker's job; before writing such recommendations, I often discuss them with the worker and occasionally with the employer.

Use of the *Guides to the Evaluation of Permanent Impairment*

The AMA's *Guides to the Evaluation of Permanent Impairment*[8] may be used to evaluate **permanent** impairment of any body system(s) from both occupational and non-occupational causes; they are not designed for use in evaluating **temporary** impairment. The *Guides* are a set of guidelines, not absolute recommendations, and are designed to bring objectivity to an area of great subjectivity by providing clinically sound and reproducible criteria useful to physicians, attorneys, and adjudicators. They espouse the philosophy that all physical and mental impairment affects the whole person: "A 95% to 100% whole-person impairment is considered to represent almost total impairment, a state that is approaching death."[8] Before using the *Guides* for evaluating cutaneous impairment, the physician should read the two introductory chapters, the glossary, and then chapter 13, "The Skin." Chapter 2, "Records and Reports," lists a suggested outline for a medical evaluation report:

1. Medical history;
2. Clinical evaluation;
3. Diagnoses;
4. Stability of the medical condition;
5. Impact of the medical condition on specific activities of daily living, including occupation;
6. Explanation for concluding that the individual is or is not likely to suffer further impairment by engaging in usual activities;
7. Explanation for concluding that accommodations or restrictions related to impairment are or are not warranted; and
8. A listing of specific impairment percentages.

The chapter on the skin lists five classes of impairment, ranging from 0% to 95% (Table 1). The impact of the disorder on the activities of daily living should be the major consideration in determining the class of impairment. The frequency and intensity of signs and symptoms and the frequency and complexity of medical treatment should guide the selection of an appropriate impairment percentage and estimate within any class.

TABLE 1. Impairment Classes and Percents for Skin Disorders*

Class 1: 0–9% Impairment	Class 2: 10–24% Impairment	Class 3: 25–54% Impairment	Class 4: 55–84% Impairment	Class 5: 85–95% Impairment
Signs and symptoms of skin disorder are present or only intermittently present;	Signs and symptoms of skin disorder are present or intermittently present;	Signs and symptoms of skin disorder are present or intermittently present;	Signs and symptoms of skin disorder are *constantly* present;	Signs and symptoms of skin disorder are *constantly* present;
and	**and**	**and**	**and**	**and**
There is no limitation or limitation in the performance of *few* activities of daily living, although exposure to certain chemical or physical agents may increase limitation temporarily.	There is limitation in the performance of *some* of the activities of daily living.	There is limitation in the performance of *many* of the activities of daily living.	There is limitation in the performance of *many* of the activities of daily living that may include intermittent confinement at home or other domicile.	There is limitation in the performance of *most* of the activities of daily living, including occasional to constant confinemnt at home or other domicile.
and	**and**	**and**	**and**	**and**
No treatment or intermittent treatment is required.	Intermittent to constant treatment may be required.	Intermittent to constant treatment may be required.	Intermittent to constant treatment may be required.	Intermittent to constant treatment may be required.

* The signs and symptoms of disorders in classes 1 and 2 may be intermittent and not present at the time of examination. The impact of the skin disorder on daily activities should be the primary consideration in determining the class of impairment. The frequency and intensity of signs and symptoms and the frequency and complexity of medical treatment should guide the selection of an appropriate impairment percentage and estimate within any class. (From Guides to the Evaluation of Permanent Impairment, 4th ed. Chicago, American Medical Association, 1993, with permission.)

The activities of daily living (ADLs) include:

1. Self-care and personal hygiene;
2. Communication;
3. Physical activity;
4. Hand functions (grasping, holding, pinching, percussive movements, and sensory discrimination);
5. Sensory function;
6. Travel;
7. Sexual function;
8. Sleep; and
9. Social and recreational activities.

Other examples of specific ADLs are listed in the glossary of the *Guides.*

The examples within each class are important guidelines for the first-time user. The fourth edition contains new examples of impairment from urticaria and skin grafts as well as refinement of some of the previous examples. Most examples are not workers' compensation cases. It is critically important to remember that impairment is not determined by diagnosis alone, but also by the effect of the disease on ADLs along with the frequency and intensity of disease and the frequency and complexity of therapy. Most cutaneous impairment falls within the first three classes, ranging from 0–54%.

Unique to the skin chapter are the discussions of pruritus, disfigurement, and scars and skin grafts. The evaluation of pruritus is based on its interference with the ADLs and the extent to which the description of pruritus is supported by objective findings, such as lichenification, excoriation, or hyperpigmentation. Disfigurement usually involves no loss of body function and little or no effect on the ADLs. Disfigurement may well impair self-image, cause lifestyle alteration, and result in social rejection. These changes are best evaluated in accordance with the criteria in the chapter on mental and behavioral conditions. Evaluation of scars and skin grafts is made according to the impact on ADLs. When impairment is based on peripheral nerve dysfunction or loss of range of motion, it may be evaluated according to the criteria in the chapters on the nervous system and musculoskeletal system.

CONCLUSIONS AND RECOMMENDATIONS

All diagnoses should be listed and summarized. A summary statement regarding causation is then made; for example, within a reasonable degree of medical certainty, the disease is or is not related to work. A physician is not required to have such an opinion and in some cases may not be able to make a determination of "probable cause." The diagnosis should include a description of specific clinical findings related to the impairment and how they relate to and compare with the criteria in the *Guides.* The impairment value also should be explained. Specific recommendations for therapy should be included, along with a brief explanation of the treatment. Recommendations for prevention, including work restrictions, are next; possible suggestions are environmental modification (e.g., exhaust ventilation, splash guards) and personal protective equipment. The effect of future exposures to chemical, physical, and biologic agents also should be addressed, along with any need for rehabilitation. Finally, the basis for the conclusions should be discussed, such as personal observations as the treating physician on specified dates, a one-time independent medical evaluation, or findings from history, old records, physical examination, and patch tests, alone or in combination. Inconsistencies and other disclaimers should be listed.[7,8]

In conclusion, evaluation of impairment is an important task for dermatologists who evaluate workers with occupational disease. Because the AMA *Guides* greatly facilitate this process, more dermatologists should become familiar with their use and application.

REFERENCES

1. American Society for Law and Medicine: Syllabus. Course on Workers' Compensation. Washington, DC, American Society for Law and Medicine, October , 1975.
2. Analysis of Workers' Compensation Laws. Washington, DC, U.S. Chamber of Commerce, 1992.
3. Centers for Disease Control: Prevalence of work disability United States, 1990. MMWR 42:757–759, 1993.
4. Centers for Disease Control: Prevalence of mobility and self-care disability—United States, 1990. MMWR 42:767–769, 1993.
5. Fisher TF: New developments in workers' compensation law. Ann NY Acad Sci 572:256–260, 1989.
6. Freeman S: Diagnosis and differential diagnosis. In Adams RM (ed): Occupational Skin Disease, 2nd ed. Philadelphia, W.B. Saunders, 1990, pp 194–214.
7. Goldstein A: Writing report letters for patients with skin disease resulting from on-the-job exposures. Dermatol Clin 2:631–641, 1984.
8. Guides to the Evaluation of Permanent Impairment, 4th ed. Chicago, American Medical Association, 1993.
9. Kane J: Selected occupational illness data by category of illness, private industry, 1992. Washington, DC, Bureau of Labor Statistics, U.S. Department of Labor, 1993 (personal communication).
10. Key M: Confusing compensation cases. Cutis 3:965–969, 1967.
11. Martin RA: Occupational Disability. Springfield, IL, Charles C Thomas, 1975.
12. Mathias CGT: Contact dermatitis and workers' compensation: Criteria for establishing occupational causation and aggravation. J Am Acad Dermatol 20:842–848, 1989.
13. Nethercott JR: Disability due to occupational contact dermatitis. Occup Med State Art Rev 1:199–203, 1986.
14. Nethercott JR: The Americans with Disabilities Act. Am J Contact Dermatitis 4:185–186, 1993.
15. Occupational injuries and illnesses in the United States by Industry, 1990. Bulletin 2399, Bureau of Labor Statistics, U.S. Department of Labor, 1992.
16. Starr J: Personal communication, September 9, 1988.

JAMES R. NETHERCOTT, MD

FITNESS TO WORK WITH SKIN DISEASE AND THE AMERICANS WITH DISABILITIES ACT OF 1990

From the Environmental and Occupational Skin Disease Center
Department of Dermatology
University of Maryland
Baltimore, Maryland

Reprint requests to:
James R. Nethercott, MD
Environmental and Occupational Skin Disease Center
Department of Dermatology
University of Maryland
405 West Redwood Street, 6th Floor
Baltimore, MD 21201

The Americans with Disabilities Act of 1990 places responsibilities on employers and workers to ensure that persons are not prevented without objective reasons from taking jobs that they can perform. The occupational physician has a difficult role in evaluating workers to determine if they have cutaneous disease that may render them unable to perform the essential job functions with reasonable accommodation and without placing the worker or others at material risk of injury or disease. Few cutaneous diseases could exclude a worker from the workplace; this chapter discusses examples of possible diseases of the skin that in certain circumstances may warrant exclusion of a prospective employee.

PROVISIONS OF THE AMERICANS WITH DISABILITIES ACT

The Americans with Disabilities Act of 1990 (ADA) came into full effect on July 26, 1992.[2,28] In contrast to the Federal Rehabilitation Act of 1973, which applied only to the federal government, federal contractors, and establishments receiving federal grants, the new act extends protection to disabled workers in the private sector. All workers except federal employees, treaty Indians, and employees of private clubs are covered by the act. Workers in the federal jurisdiction continue to be protected under the Rehabilitation Act of 1973.

The law places a general duty on the employer to allow a prospective employee to engage in a job if she or he is able to perform the *"essential components"* of the job without putting other workers at risk or placing her- or himself at *"material risk of harm."* In addition, the new law requires that the employer make *"reasonable accommodations"* in the work tasks and environment to allow a prospective employee to perform the essential components of the job. The term "reasonable" is not completely defined at this time; the definition will be established through precedent as the law is applied.

An employer no longer can require a medical examination of a prospective employee before offering employment. A single exception is specifically made: a urine test to screen for drugs of abuse.

Once an employment offer has been made, the prospective employee may be required to submit to a medical examination, but the criteria that can be used to determine whether a prospective worker is fit to perform the essential components of the job are restricted. The employer may not exclude a worker on the basis of past drug addiction if he or she has been or is in treatment. Paternalistic reasons may not be used as a basis for excluding a person from a job as long as the person can perform the essential job functions (EJFs) with reasonable accommodation. In other words, even if the employer or his or her agent (e.g., physician, nurse, physiotherapist, psychologist) believes that a worker is likely to be placed at increased risk of an adverse health outcome, the worker cannot be excluded. To exclude a worker, one must establish that the job will place the worker or others at material risk to health. It is not enough to have reason to believe that the job at some later date may aggravate a preexisting condition or place the worker at increased risk of developing a chronic disease at some distant time. The basis for exclusion must be known to be a valid predictor of health risk for the worker in question or his or her fellow workers.

Workers have to establish that they have the educational background, experience, skills, licenses, and any other job related qualification standards and that they are able to perform the tasks essential to the job, with or without reasonable accommodation.

Employers must be able to establish that the prospective worker cannot perform the EJFs even with reasonable accommodation to deny the job. To make such a determination, the employer must carefully examine each job to determine its EJFs, which must be updated constantly and current at the time of evaluation of a prospective applicant. The employer must take several parameters into consideration when determining whether a given function is an EJF. The factors to be considered include: whether the purpose of the position is to perform the specific function, the number of other employees available who are capable of performing the function or among whom the performance of the function can be distributed, and the degree of expertise or skill required to perform the function. These criteria can be established by the creation of precise, complete job descriptions prepared and written before advertising or interviewing for a job. This process entails evaluating the work experience of present and/or past employees in the job, the time spent performing each EJF, the consequences of not requiring that an employee perform a given EJF, and the terms of the collective bargaining agreement that controls the work contract in a given place of employment.

The employer has the sole responsibility of determining whether an adjustment in the workplace to accommodate a worker can be made. The employer has the sole right to manage under the employment contract except as modified by the act or other state or federal legislation or by terms set forth in a collective agreement with the union. The employer also has sole discretion with respect to the allocation of monies to modify the workplace or to provide special equipment. At his or her discretion, based on the above factors, the manager has to decide if what is needed to assist a given disabled person can be reasonably provided, with the knowledge that a prospective worker who disagrees has the right to seek redress through the Equal Employment Opportunities Commission (EEOC). The EEOC has produced a technical manual[6] to assist managers in making such decisions. The manual provides examples of situations wherein the commission believes that certain decisions with respect to accommodation would be reasonable. Physicians can obtain a copy of the manual from the EEOC at no charge simply by calling the commission in Washington, DC, and requesting that a copy be mailed.

It is essential that the examining physician who performs a preplacement examination after the offer of a job have full disclosure of the EJFs of the position that the worker has been offered. The physician must be able to relate the abilities of the prospective worker to the demands of the position. The role of the physician in this capacity is not straightforward. To establish that a condition poses a direct threat may be straightforward in a few instances (e.g., tunnel vision in a worker operating a forklift truck), but in most instances valid information to allow prediction of a disabled worker's risk to self or others is simply not available. As mentioned above, paternalism is specifically barred; thus, even though an examining physician may believe that the proposed job increases the worker's risk of developing a medical condition (e.g., an ulcer of the foot in a diabetic worker), neither the doctor nor the employer has the right to deny the job unless they are able to quantify the risk and establish that it may result in material harm. Such determinations necessitate considerable discretion. This chapter provides the reader with some guidance as to how skin diseases may be approached.

EXCLUSION OF WORKERS WITH SKIN DISEASE

Only a few skin diseases constitute a basis for excluding a prospective employee.

Cutaneous Infections

Infectious diseases certainly may be a basis for exclusion, including the following:

Herpes Simplex Virus. If a health care professional experiences a recurrent herpetic whitlow of a finger due to herpes simplex virus, he or she would pose a risk to patients if direct patient contact was an EJF.[4] If it is not possible to suppress the disease fully with medical therapy and if the job is such that patient contact cannot reasonably be managed by others during attacks of herpes infection, the disease constitutes a bona fide criterion for exclusion.

Dermatophytes. One may consider excluding a person with chronic tinea infection of the hands resistant to treatment if a job involves extensive skin contact, such as a masseur whose clients may be placed at risk. Human experimental studies[15] indicate that large inocula are needed to induce dermatophyte infections. A break in the skin or the tight occlusion of a bandage on footwear, combined with inoculation, are likely requirements for the exposed person to contract the infection. Although transmission may be possible, it is quite unlikely. Thus, while one may consider the risk of dermatophyte transmission, the outcome (i.e., tinea) and the chances of transmission do not favor exclusion of an infected person from a job involving contact with others' skin. On the other hand, a carrier may be required to wear protective equipment (e.g., gloves) when working.

Pyogenic Cocci. Recurrent impetigo of the face or hands poses an unacceptable risk to others in a person preparing food that can be inoculated and possibly lead to staphylococcal food poisoning. Similarly, a person who was performing surgery or assisting at surgery may pose a risk to patients if he or she were carrying staphylococci in the nares. Any person with chronic dermatoses (e.g., psoriasis, atopic dermatitis) is more likely to grow pyogenic cocci on affected skin than normal persons and thus may pose a risk in close contact with compromised patients in a hospital. It seems reasonable to exclude carriers from certain hospital settings (e.g., operating room, postoperative nursing, immunologically suppressed patients) if they are shown chronically to carry virulent organisms on their skin.

Eczematous Dermatitis

Eczematous skin facilitates the growth of more virulent organisms (e.g., staphylococci, streptococci) that may lead to overt impetiginization or be found only on skin culture. Carriers with involvement of exposed skin surfaces may pose a risk to others in certain personal service occupations with close skin-to-skin contact.

Chronic dermatitides affecting the hand may limit grip strength, and for positions in which grip strength has been quantified as an EJF, a person with chronic eczematous dermatitis of the hand may well be unable to meet the objective job requirements. Such individuals also may have to apply to their skin topical agents that reduce frictional resistance and thus the ability to grasp objects. This may be a significant problem in a job in which such ability is essential, such as driving heavy machinery.

Dermatoses of the Feet

Foot dermatoses such as chronic tinea pedis, psoriasis, eczematous dermatitis, recurrent bullous eruption of the hands and feet, and epidermolysis bullosa or even callosities of the feet may be severe enough to limit the person's ability to walk for long periods or to run. In occupations in which these tasks are essential (e.g., police work, fire-fighting) the affected person may well be unable to perform EJFs, such as running a certain distance at a given speed. Such limitations may preclude the person's ability to perform the job.

Skin Disease Affecting Thermoregulation

Anhidrotic ectodermal dysplasia is a rare skin disease in which the individual lacks eccrine sweat ducts. Such individuals are not able to work in conditions of prolonged heat stress because of their inability to sweat as a thermoregulatory mechanism. Such jobs and such patients are uncommon.

Patients with chronic erythroderma also pose problems of response in extremely cold outdoor jobs, because they would be susceptible to cold injury and hypothermia. It may be reasonable to exclude affected individuals from jobs involving a risk of prolonged periods of exposure to cold because of the risk of fatal outcome or severe disability.

Physical Agent Intolerance

Certain skin disorders are associated with increased response to ultraviolet light, such as lupus erythematosus, persistent light reaction, and solar urticaria. Affected individuals probably would be unable to perform the EJFs of a job involving extensive outdoor work in the sunlight unless they were photoprotected; for severe cases, even a sunscreen may not be adequate. In certain instances the cause of photosensitivity is known (e.g., the light-sensitive porphyrias, lupus erythematosus), and specific therapy is available. For many persons, however, the underlying process is idiopathic and only avoidance of exposure or use of photoprotection is of value. Direct exposure to sunlight would be expected to exacerbate their disease to an extent that they would be unable to continue to work. A trial of work exposure may be necessary to determine the level of impairment and whether it is compatible with performing the EJFs of the job.

Similarly, persons with Raynaud's disease are susceptible to cold, and if the disease is severe, they may be at risk of developing gangrene of the fingers with prolonged cold exposure. A similar risk applies to scleroderma of the acrosclerotic type, which is characterized by peripheral vasospasm in response to cold. The ability to accommodate the worker is crucial in such situations. If it is impossible to avoid prolonged cold exposure in the context of the job and if reliable personal protective devices cannot be provided, exclusion is justified.

Cold urticaria is another disorder that may make outdoor work in cold environments impossible. Severely affected persons may develop marked angioedema on exposure to cold and thus be unable to perform manual activity. In certain jobs, therefore, the disorder may be a basis for exclusion.

WORK-AGGRAVATED SKIN DISEASES THAT MAY REQUIRE ACCOMMODATION

A number of skin diseases are known to be made worse by certain work exposures, but the aggravation would not be expected to interfere materially with the worker's ability to perform the EJFs.

Psoriasis and Lichen Planus

Psoriasis affects 1% of the American population.[18] Some affected individuals develop new psoriatic lesions at sites of physical injury, such as cuts and chemical or thermal burns; this tendency is known as the Koebner phenomenon. According to a study by Eyre and Kreuger,[7] 30–50% of psoriatic patients report developing new lesions at sites of trauma. In another study by the same authors, however, only 5–10% of psoriatic patients made such an association.[16] Such persons, if engaged in physically hazardous work (e.g., arc welding) may develop new psoriatic lesions at sites of cutaneous injury. The frequency of such responses is variable, and probably less than one-half of psoriatic patients experience this phenomenon. Although not a life-threatening matter, new lesions usually persist and thus accumulate over the years of service. In some states such disease is compensable; even so, under the new law, the employer would not have the right to exclude an affected worker from employment. There is no basis for exclusion in psoriasis for two reasons: (1) occurrence of the Koebner phenomenon, is unpredictable, and (2) even if such a response occurs, it may not impair the worker's ability to perform the EJFs.

The same situation applies to lichen planus, a less common disease than psoriasis, which affects 4.4/1000 outpatients in the United States.[3] Lichen planus also may erupt at sites of injury, but the phenomenon is not as striking as in psoriasis. The frequency of the phenomenon in patients with lichen planus is unknown, but it is likely less than in patients with psoriasis. The same considerations apply to this disease as to psoriasis in terms of fitness to work under the new act.

Vitiligo

Vitiligo is a depigmenting skin disease that also develops at sites of cutaneous injury in about one-third of affected persons.[20] It may be quite disfiguring cosmetically, but it does not impair the worker's ability to perform EJFs and thus does not qualify as a basis for exclusion.

Endogenous Eczematous Dermatitis

Constitutional eczema may be aggravated by physical injury and exposure to irritants. Many studies link atopic dermatitis with work-related hand dermatitis.[9,17,25-27] The disease typically begins in childhood in association with hay fever and asthma, which predispose to the development of hand dermatitis during wet work or exposure to irritants.[18] The disease was shown to affect 7/1,000 Americans in the NHANES study.[12] The risk of hand dermatitis increases significantly in affected persons who do wet work; in some circumstances the risk is possibly as high as 50%. It is unlikely, however, that a personal history of atopic dermatitis at the time of a preplacement examination would constitute an adequate basis for exclusion for two reasons: (1) the development of hand dermatitis would not necessarily interfere with the worker's ability to perform the EJFs, and (2) history alone does not guarantee that the worker will become so affected. The examining physician, nonetheless, may counsel the prospective employee about the risk of developing hand dermatitis and suggest that taking the job may be ill advised.

The other common eczematous dermatitis posing a work-related problem is dyshidrotic eczema. In her seminal investigation of hand dermatitis in Sweden, Agrup[1] found that this common disorder accounted for 6% of cases. The disease is characterized by vesicular eruption on the palms, soles, or both; it follows a relapsing course and is aggravated by exposure to irritants. Although occasionally the disease is severe enough to make manual work or walking difficult and thus to result in temporary disability in certain occupations, it is usually only a nuisance. Dyshidrotic eczema is capricious and may exacerbate and remit for no apparent reason. The uncertainty of the disease makes impossible the extrapolation of impairment; thus, exclusion from a position on this basis is equally nonfeasible.

Contact Dermatitis

Contact dermatitis often affects the hands, especially in work-related cases. Once it develops on the hands, it often becomes chronic.[5,22] Many studies have indicated the poor prognosis in such individuals, who often develop persistent skin disease of the hands for many years.[10,21,24,29,30] Affected individuals often do not improve if they change occupation, unless a specific insular allergic contactant accounts for the problem.[19,23] For the majority, the disease persists, and accommodation, such as personal protective equipment and avoidance of defined exposures, is probably the best method to control skin disease. Education of both the affected person and his or her coworkers is important to ensure understanding of the problem and acceptance of its chronicity. Accommodation ameliorates the disease, and the person remains gainfully employed.[11,13,19,23] The reasonableness of such accommodation, judged on the basis of the criteria outlined above, determines whether the worker continues at the job.

ADVANTAGES OF THE AMERICANS WITH DISABILITIES ACT FOR THE WORKER WITH SKIN DISEASE

Prospective employees with skin disease have been at a competitive disadvantage when applying for work, because skin disease is visible and easily labels them as "sick." Although people with a chronic skin condition may be perfectly able to perform the EJFs, in the past they often were excluded on the basis that they would not be able to do so. This at times paternalistic exclusion has had adverse social consequences in many instances.[14] The Americans with Disabilities Act requires that an employer provide reasonable proof that the worker cannot perform the EJFs before employment can be denied. Furthermore, many workers with chronic hand eczema have found it difficult to persuade a present or prospective employer to provide simple personal protective equipment that would allow them to perform the job. The provision of such equipment is now no longer optional but almost certainly will be considered a reasonable accommodation.

Workers who previously have been denied return to work because of a chronic skin disease, whether work-related or not, need to recognize that the new law to some degree empowers them to seek return to work with suitable accommodation.

Both the personal physician and the occupational physician are in a position to help such workers to obtain reasonable accommodation and to encourage them and their fellow workers to accept the accommodation as an opportunity for continued gainful employment.

CONCLUSIONS

Few instances of skin disease preclude a person from performing a given job, although a specific skin disorder may be considered a basis for exclusion in certain circumstances. The Americans with Disabilities Act is important, because it discourages employers from denying work to persons with skin disease as long as they are able to do the job. In due course employers and coworkers will recognize that most individuals with a chronic skin condition can perform normal work activities, particularly with support and encouragement both at work and at home. A decision to dismiss such workers must take into consideration the poor prospects for reemployment once they leave the firm at which the skin disease developed, regardless of whether the disease is work-related. Such workers are often remarkable contributors and exemplary employees. They have to be well-motivated, positive persons to tolerate the skin disease and continue to work.

REFERENCES

1. Agrup G: Hand eczema and hand dermatoses in south Sweden. Acta Derm Venereol 49(Suppl 61):1–132, 1969.
2. Anfield R: American with Disabilities Act of 1990: A primer of title I provisions for occupational health care professionals. J Occup Med 34:503–509, 1992.
3. Arndt K, Lichen P: In Fitzpatrick T, Eisen A, Wolff K, et al (eds): Dermatology in General Medicine, 4th ed. New York, McGraw-Hill, 1993, p 1134.
4. Crumpacker C, Gulick R: Herpes simplex. In Fitzpatrick T, Eisen A, Wolff K, et al (eds): Dermatology in General Medicine, 4th ed. New York, McGraw-Hill, 1993, pp 2536–2537.
5. Edman B: Sites of contact dermatitis in relationship to particular allergens. Contact Dermatitis 13:129–135, 1985.
6. Equal Employment Opportunities Commission: Technical Manual for the Americans with Disabilities Act of 1990. Washington, DC, Equal Employment Opportunities Commission, 1991.
7. Eyre R, Kreuger G: The Koebner Response in psoriasis. In Roenigh H, Maibach H (eds): Psoriasis. New York, Marcel Dekker, 1984, pp 34–38.

8. Farber E, Nall M: The natural history of psoriasis in 5600 patients. Dermatologica 148:1–18, 1974.
9. Forsbeck M, Skog E, Asbrink E: Atopic hand dermatitis: A comparison with atopic dermatitis without hand improvement, especially with respect to influence of work and development of contact sensitization. Acta Derm Venereol (Stockh) 63:9–13, 1983.
10. Hogan D, Dannaker C, Maibach H: The prognosis of contact dermatitis. J Am Acad Dermatol 23:300–307, 1990.
11. Holness D, Nethercott J: Is a worker's understanding of their diagnosis an important determinant of outcome in occupational contact dermatitis? Contact Dermatitis 25:296–301, 1991.
12. Johnson M: Prevalence of dermatologic disease among persons 1–74 years of age: United States. In Advance Data from Vital and Health Statistics of the National Center for Health Statistics, no. 4, January 26, 1977.
13. Jowett S, Ryan T: Skin disease and handicap: An analysis of the impact of skin conditions. Soc Sci Med 20:425–429, 1985.
14. Keczkes K, Bhate S, Wyatt E: The outcome of primary irritant contact dermatitis. Br J Dermatol 109:665–668, 1983.
15. Knight A: A review of experimental human fungus infections. J Invest Dermatol 197:1017–1020, 1972.
16. Kreuger C, Eyre R: Trigger actors in psoriasis. Dermatol Clin 373–378, 1985.
17. Lammintausta K, Kalimo K, Aantaa S: Course of hand dermatitis in hospital workers. Contact Dermatitis 8:327–332, 1982.
18. Leung D, Rhodes A, Geha R, et al: Atopic dermatitis. In Fitzpatrick T, Eisen A, Wolff K, et al (eds): Dermatology in General Medicine, 4th ed. New York, McGraw-Hill, 1993, pp 1543–1564.
19. Morris G: "Why doesn't the worker's skin clear up"? Arch Ind Hyg 10:43–49, 1954.
20. Mosher D, Fitzpatrick T, Hori Y, Ortonne J-P: Disorders of pigmentation. In Fitzpatrick T, Eisen A, Wolff K, et al (eds): Dermatology in General Medicine, 4th ed. New York, McGraw-Hill, 1993, p 924.
21. Nethercott J, Gallant C: Disability due to occupational contact dermatitis. Occup Med State Art Rev 1:199–203, 1986.
22. Nethercott J, Holness DL, Adams R, et al: Patch testing with a routine screening tray in North America, 1985–1989. IV: Occupation of response. Am J Contact Dermatitis (in press).
23. O'Quinn S, Cole J, Many H: Problems of disability and rehabilitation in patients with chronic skin diseases. Arch Dermatol 105:35–41, 1972.
24. Rosen R, Freeman S: Prognosis of occupational contact dermatitis in New South Wales, Australia. Contact Dermatitis 29:88–93, 1993.
25. Rystedt I: Hand eczema and long-term prognosis in atopic dermatitis. Acta Derm Venereol (Stockh) 117(Suppl):1–59, 1985.
26. Rystedt I: Long-term follow-up in atopic dermatitis. Acta Derm Venereol (Stockh) 114(Suppl):117–120, 1985.
27. Shmunes E, Keil JE: Role of atopy in occupational dermatosis. Contact Dermatitis 11:174–178, 1984.
28. St. Clair S, Shults T: American with Disabilities Act: Considerations for the practice of occupational medicine. J Occup Med 34:510–517, 1992.
29. Vestey J, Gawkrodger, Wong W, Buxton P: Analysis of 501 consecutive contact clinic consultations. Contact Dermatitis 15:119–125, 1986.
30. Wall L, Gebauer K: Occupational skin disease in Western Australia. Contact Dermatitis 24:101–109, 1991.

JERRY E. COOLEY, MD
JAMES R. NETHERCOTT, MD

PROGNOSIS OF OCCUPATIONAL SKIN DISEASE

From the Environmental and Occupational Skin Disease Center
Department of Dermatology
University of Maryland
Baltimore, Maryland

Reprint requests to:
James R. Nethercott, MD
Environmental and Occupational Skin Disease Center
Department of Dermatology
University of Maryland
405 West Redwood Street, 6th Floor
Baltimore, MD 21201

The prognosis in occupational skin disease (OSD), which is largely irritant (ICD) and allergic contact dermatitis (ACD), is guarded. Many investigations over the last five decades have documented that a large proportion of workers developing such disease do not improve with present methods of secondary preventive intervention and treatment. Although cases of ACD may do better when a specific cause can be found and avoided, ACD due to the metals nickel and chromium has a poor prognosis. Job changes are of equivocal value. Early diagnosis and intervention are associated with a better prognosis for cure. Medical management alone has not modified the outcome significantly over the last decade. Greater attention to primary prevention through regulation of exposure to irritants and sensitizers, combined with more effective measures for control of industrial hygiene, offers the possibility of more effective management.

COMPENSATION CLAIMS IN THE UNITED STATES

Data from the Bureau of Labor Statistics (BLS) indicate that occupational contact dermatitis (OCD) accounts for about 20% of work-related disease for which compensation claims were paid in the early 1980s.[17] In 1982 the incidence was 0.7 cases per 1,000 full-time workers in the United States.[17] This estimate probably underrepresents significantly the true extent of such disease in the American workplace because of underreporting and factors mitigating against successful claims, which form the basis for the statistic. In the early 1970s the proportion of paid claims for skin disease was even higher—about 30%. This decline may not indicate a lower incidence of work-related skin disease but rather changes in reporting the data to the BLS; for example, more skin disease may have been treated as first-aid rather than lost-time claims. In addition, work-related orthopedic disease, in particular cumulative trauma disorders, have increased substantially as a basis for compensation claims and thus reduced the relative proportion of claims related to skin disease. In any case, skin disease remains an important public health problem in the American workplace. There is reason to question whether the situation is improving despite the decline in the proportion of paid compensation claims reported.

The present chapter reviews the prognosis in work-related skin disease, which consists largely of OCD. Because of its prevalence, OCD has enormous medical, social, and economic consequences in the American workplace.[1] Health-care providers face much confusion when confronted by affected patients; for example, whether a change of jobs or assiduous avoidance of the suspected cutaneous toxicant will improve the skin condition is often not as clear as it may seem. Recent research on the prognosis of OCD has uncovered important factors relevant to the clinician. This chapter updates the 1986 review by Nethercott and Gallant,[19] which was published in this journal.

PREVALENCE OF OCCUPATIONAL SKIN DISEASE

Rather than rely on data derived from paid compensation claims, one can examine the prevalence of skin disease in given populations of workers. This method gives a different measure of frequency, because it identifies not only compensable disease but also workers who have not come forward to seek medical attention or compensation. On the other hand, because it is a cross-sectional method, persons with severe disease, compensated or not, who either are too sick to work or have left the workplace will not be accounted for. Several investigators have examined selected populations of workers. Swedish investigators studying occupational dermatitis in construction workers found a prevalence of 7.4% among 365 workers in one study[25] and of 18% among 1,071 workers in another.[28] A study of 2,239 house painters[13] found a prevalence of 3.9%. Such estimates of point prevalence cannot be compared directly with the 1985 incident rate of 0.7/1,000 full-time workers in the United States, but they do suggest either that the American data represent a significant underestimation (possibly for the reasons discussed above) or that the incident rate in the studied occupations is significantly higher, at least in terms of observable as opposed to compensable disease. Even if American workers remained in their trade for 30 years and had disease from the onset of employment, the prevalence at a given point in time would not reach the levels reported among construction workers in Sweden if the incidence rate were comparable to the BLS figure. Numerous caveats, of course, must be taken into consideration. Prospective data are needed to address the matter formally. Two points, nonetheless, are clear: (1) skin dysfunction is relatively common, and (2) it is not found with uniform frequency among different occupations.

NATURAL HISTORY OF OCCUPATIONAL CONTACT DERMATITIS

Work-related skin disease may begin at any age, occasionally even in the sixth decade.[6] Often this condition begins in the middle years of life.[20] Halbert et al.[11]

reported that the median age of onset of occupational ACD due to chromium was 34 years in their study population of Australian workers and that 61% of patients were younger than 40 years. The same group of investigators reported that of 993 patients with occupational dermatoses evaluated in Western Australia, 75% were less than 40 years old at onset of their disease.[29] Thus OCD affects workers at all ages but in certain instances, including chromium allergy, seems to begin earlier. Nethercott and Holness found that OCD tends to occur in hairdressers after only a few years of employment.[14]

OUTCOME IN OCCUPATIONAL CONTACT DERMATITIS

It has been known for a long time that in general patients with work-related dermatitis have a poor prognosis for clearing of their condition. In 1938 Mayr reported that 32% of 301 workers still had active dermatitis after 10 years of follow-up.[18] In a follow-up of a cohort of compensated chromium-sensitive workers in Northern Ireland, Burrows[3] found that over 70% still had problems with skin disease 10 years after it first developed. Fregert[10] also found a persistence of disease in Danish workers followed for 10 years after initial diagnosis. Cronin[7] found persistent dermatitis in 75% of 32 catering workers, most of whom were followed for longer than 2 years. Schubert et al.[26] reported that 35% of 104 nickel-allergic patients followed for 3 years still had active disease. Dannaker et al.[8] followed 12 patients with ACD due to chromium for up to 24 years and found that 67% were still affected. Three more recent investigations have examined the rate of persistent disease in workers with OCD. In a Canadian study, Holness and Nethercott[15] followed patients evaluated at an occupational dermatology clinic and found that 4 of 10 had persistent disease, although 70% of patients with persistent disease reported improvement. In 1991 Wall and Gebauer[29] reported a landmark investigation based on compensation files of Australian workers. Follow-up was almost complete. The authors once again demonstrated that a significant proportion of compensated workers had persistent disease years after onset. In 1993 Rosen and Freeman[22] reported a rate of persistent disease at follow-up among workers in New South Wales that was similar to the rate reported by Holness and Nethercott in Canada.

In summary, after more than 50 years of observation and investigation in many parts of the world, it is clear that OCD tends to be associated with at best a guarded prognosis. Although the studies are not entirely comparable because of variations in methods and length of follow-up, basis for case-finding, and proportion of potential patients actually followed in the identified population, no evidence indicates that the outcome has improved significantly over the past five decades.

RISK FACTORS AFFECTING OUTCOME IN OCCUPATIONAL CONTACT DERMATITIS

Many studies have tried to identify characteristics that may be associated with a better or worse prognosis in OCD.

One of the strongest predictors of future disease is a history of chronic dermatitis.[1,12] The longer the person has had dermatitis before seeking treatment and initiating intervention, the worse the outlook for complete resolution of disease. For instance, Halbert et al.[11] found that the only significant predictor of chronicity among 33 patients who had changed jobs but continued to have active dermatitis was the presence of symptoms for more than 12 months. These findings echo similar observations by Chan-Yeung et al.[4] in workers with western red cedar asthma. The most important predictor of outcome was the length of time the worker persisted with exposure after onset of asthma. These findings underscore the importance of early diagnosis and intervention as a method to mitigate against the development of severe and chronic OCD.

The particular contactant initiating OCD may also be an important determinant of prognosis. Oil products, plastics (e.g., epoxy resins, amine curing agents, acrylic monomers), and rubber additives tend to be less likely to produce chronic disease. This observation may be due to the fact that affected workers are better able to avoid the specific contactant to which they have become sensitized. In contrast, nickel and chromium are associated with a poor prognosis.[2,3,5,8,19] In keeping with this difference, Rosen and Freeman[22] recently reported that patients with ACD due to p-phenylenediamine had a much better prognosis than patients with ACD due to chromium: 90% vs. 41%, respectively, improved at follow-up between 1 and 5 years after onset of ACD. The same authors found no significant difference in prognosis in ACD and ICD. Holness and Nethercott,[15] on the other hand, found that patients with ACD fared better than patients with ICD; patient understanding of the disease, however, was an important predictor of outcome.

Schmunes and Keil[27] concluded from a study of compensation cases in South Carolina that workers with atopy were more likely to develop OCD and that they tended to fare worse than nonatopic workers. Forsbeck et al.[9] found that workers with atopic dermatitis (AD) were likely to develop OCD but that they improved with control of exposure to irritants. In a retrospective/prospective study, Rystedt[23,24] found that children with AD evaluated at the Karolinska Institute were at considerably greater risk of developing hand dermatitis if they took occupations involving wet work than individuals without AD. This difference was not evident in patients who had only mucosal allergy rather than AD. Rosen and Freeman[22] reported that 79% of workers without AD improved over a period of follow-up compared with 62.4% of workers with AD. Holness and Nethercott[14] also found that workers with both AD and OCD were more likely to have persistent disease and less likely to improve than workers with OCD alone. Workers with both conditions, however, lost less time from work and were less likely to have filed a worker's compensation claim than other workers followed in Canada.

THE EFFECT OF A CHANGE IN OCCUPATION

Workers, employers, worker's compensation carriers, and physicians often assume that a change of occupation will result in clearing of the dermatitis. However, there is evidence to the contrary. Keczkes et al.[16] found no difference in clearance of dermatitis between 64 workers with ICD who left their jobs and 124 who stayed. In a study of chromium dermatitis, Halbert et al.[11] reported that 89% of 62 workers who remained at their jobs continued to be affected compared with 69% of 58 workers who left their job because of skin disease yet remained affected. The second group, however, contained 7 workers who had further exposure to chromium at their new job, leaving 33 workers for whom change of job did not solve the problem. Although advising the worker to leave the job may seem like the obvious and best solution, it often is not. The employer most likely to accommodate a worker with a skin disability is often the employer for whom he has been working. A job change, unless it means complete avoidance of a specific allergen such as epoxy resin, is almost inevitably associated with continuing skin disease that may impair the worker's ability to retain the next job. Furthermore, skin disease is an obvious impediment that may bias an employer from hiring the worker in the first place. The support and continued management of skin disease while the worker continues to be exposed poses a highly significant challenge for the worker, his or her superiors, and the health-care provider.[21]

Holness and Nethercott[15] found that a worker's understanding of the diagnosis is associated with the course of disease. Only 33% of 230 workers could recall accurately whether the diagnosis was allergic or irritant contact dermatitis. Those who recalled the wrong diagnosis were twice as likely to have dermatitis that was still active as well as more severe; those who had no idea of the diagnosis were three times as likely to have the same problems. This study suggests that patient education is essential to improving outcome.

Finally, the research methodology used to measure disease outcome can have an effect on how it is reported. Traditionally, outcome was measured on a two-dimensional scale: symptomatic versus asymptomatic. Using a graded 5-point scale, Rosen and Freeman[22] were able to document over time significant improvements in OCD that would not have appeared significant with the traditional method.

CONCLUSION

OCD continues to be a pressing public health problem in the workplace. New evidence further substantiates the guarded prognosis. It is clear that for some contactants, identification and avoidance of further exposure, especially if carried out early in the course of disease, are associated with a favorable outcome. It is equally clear that in many instances the differentiation between ICD and ACD is difficult and possibly of no great importance, because workers tend to do poorly with either diagnosis. The hope, supported by a few studies, is that specific identification may modify the outlook somewhat. In cases of ICD that have been established for some time, the best approach is probably to support the patient, to counsel him or her to remain at the job, and to do what is possible to seek accommodation under the terms of the Americans with Disabilities Act of 1990. A job change is unlikely to lead to clearing of the disease.

Primary prevention is the obvious answer to the problem; secondary and tertiary preventive measures have not proved particularly effective. Primary prevention involves developing standards for exposure to known irritants and sensitizers that can be monitored and enforced. Such standards are forthcoming. Recent work related to the release of rubber accelerators from gloves and Danish legislation limiting the commerce of products releasing metal that may come in contact with the skin are a step in this direction. Better evaluation of protective equipment to ensure its efficacy is also needed. Without significant advances in both measurement of exposure and legislation to limit exposure, the problem is likely to continue, and the prognosis is likely to remain poor.

REFERENCES

1. Agrup G: Hand eczema and other hand dermatoses in South Sweden. Acta Derm Venereol (Stockh) 49:61–90, 1969.
2. Breit R, Turk RBM: The medical and social fate of the dichromate allergic patient. Br J Dermatol 94:349–351, 1976.
3. Burrows D: Prognosis in industrial dermatitis. Br J Dermatol 87:145–148, 1972.
4. Chan-Yeung M: Natural history of occupational asthma: Relevance of type of agent and other factors in the rate of development of symptoms in affected subjects. J Allergy Clin Immunol 90:937–944, 1992.

5. Christensen OB: Prognosis in nickel allergy and hand eczema. Contact Dermatitis 8:7–15, 1982.
6. Coenraads P, Nater J: Sickness and disease from work due to skin diseases in the construction industry: Review of the literature. Dermatosen 32:17–21, 1984.
7. Cronin E: Dermatitis of the hands in caterers. Contact Dermatitis 17:265–269, 1987.
8. Dannaker DJ, White IR, Rycroft RJG: Long-term prognosis in occupational chromate allergy: An 18 year follow-up study. Contact Dermatitis 21:59, 1989.
9. Forsbeck M, Skog E, Asbrink E: Atopic hand dermatitis: A comparison with atopic dermatitis without hand improvement, especially with respect to influence of work and development of contact sensitization. Acta Derm Venereol 63:9–13, 1983.
10. Fregert S: Occupational dermatitis in a 10-year material. Contact Dermatitis 1:96–107, 1975.
11. Halbert A, Gebauer K, Wall L: Prognosis of occupational chromate dermatitis. Contact Dermatitis 27:214–220, 1992.
12. Hogan DJ, Dannaker CJ, Maibach HI: The prognosis of contact dermatitis. J Am Acad Dermatol 23:300–307, 1990.
13. Hogberg M, Wahlberg J: Health screening for occupational dermatoses in house painters. Contact Dermatitis 100–106, 1980.
14. Holness D, Nethercott J: Dermatitis in hairdressers. Dermatol Clin 8:119–126, 1990.
15. Holness DL, Nethercott JR: Is a worker's understanding of their diagnosis an important determinant of outcome in occupational contact dermatitis? Contact Dermatitis 25:296–301, 1991.
16. Keczkes K, Bhate SM, Wyatt E: The outcome of primary irritant hand dermatitis. Br J Dermatol 109:665–669, 1983.
17. Mathias C: The cost of occupational skin disease. Arch Dermatol 121:332–334, 1985.
18. Mayr J: Uber das Schicksal von 300 Ekzematikern. Arch Dermatol Syphilol 177:83–89, 1938.
19. Nethercott J, Gallant C: Disability due to occupational contact dermatitis. Occup Med State Art Rev 1:99–203, 1986.
20. Nethercott J, Holness D, Adams R, Belsito D, et al: Patch testing with a routine screening tray in North America, 1985–1989. IV: Occupation of response. Am J Contact Dermatitis (in press).
21. O'Quinn SE, Cole J, Many H: Problems of disability and rehabilitation in patients with chronic skin diseases. Arch Dermatol 105:35–41, 1972.
22. Rosen RH, Freeman S: Prognosis of occupational contact dermatitis in New South Wales, Australia. Contact Dermatitis 29:88–93, 1993.
23. Rystedt I: Hand eczema and long-term prognosis in atopic dermatitis. Acta Derm Venereol (Stockh) 117(Suppl):1–59, 1985.
24. Rystedt I: Long term follow-up in atopic dermatitis. Acta Derm Venereol (Stockh) 114(Suppl):117–120, 1985.
25. Schaulow I, Minkow D, Dessew D: Berufs Dermatosen 13:276–283, 1965.
26. Schubert H, Berova N, Czernielewski A, et al: Epidemiology of nickel allergy. Contact Dermatitis 16:122–130, 1987.
27. Shmunes E, Keil JE: Role of atopy in occupational dermatosis. Contact Dermatitis 11:174–178, 1984.
28. Wahlberg J: Health screening for occupational skin diseases in building workers. Berufs Dermatosen 17:184–198, 1969.
29. Wall L, Gebauer K: Occupational skin disease in Western Australia. Contact Dermatitis 24:101–109, 1991.

J. B. ROSS, MB, BS, FRCPC, DObstRCOG

WORKERS' COMPENSATION FOR SKIN DISEASE

Professor of Medicine
(Dermatology)
Dalhousie University
Halifax, Nova Scotia

Reprint requests to:
Dr. J. Barrie Ross
Room 4-198 ACC
Victoria General Hospital
Halifax, NS B3H 2Y9

Workers' compensation is "a social welfare program through which employers bear some of the cost of employment injuries and occupational disease experienced by their employees."[9] Patients are encountered in practice every day who have work-related illness. One third of the lives of all patients is spent in productive work. The cost of skin disease related to work is among the highest of occupational diseases when considered on an individual basis.[21] Thus patients who have work-related skin disease must be identified and managed. An important part of that care consists of dealing with compensation for the disorder and the public bodies that deal with it. Most countries have enacted national or regional legislation covering workers' compensation, and practitioners should be aware of the relevant local regulations. This chapter summarizes important principles in relation to work-caused dermatosis and its compensation management.

HISTORICAL BACKGROUND

Ramazzini[10,13] (1633–1714), a teacher in northern Italy, wrote the first account of trade diseases. The study of trade diseases was taken up "in order that workers could earn their living without bodily injury." In earlier times, the only recourse that existed for compensation for work-related injury was under common law. Ancient sources contain many references to this process.[25] However, under common law, most frequently the worker's injury has not been due to willful, malicious, or neglectful damage. That type of damage is the province of tort law. Tort law is "concerned with the prevention of or compensation for harm sustained by a person through the unlawful or dangerous activity of others."[8] As it became difficult and expensive for workers to obtain redress under the common law system, there was increasing pressure for protective social welfare legislation in the mid-19th century.

The first of modern forms of comprehensive social insurance legislation to correct this situation, including redress for work injuries, was introduced by Bismarck in Germany in 1884.[17] It was followed by similar legislation enacted in the United Kingdom during the next decade. Adoption in North America took place somewhat later, in the early part of the 20th century. The United States initially passed Employers' Liability Acts in 1908 and 1909, followed by workers' compensation legislation starting in 1910. In Canada, Sir William Meredith was commissioned to undertake a study that culminated as the Ontario Workers' Compensation Legislation in 1914, becoming effective in 1915. Initially there were a variety of programs varying from compulsory social insurance to an obligation to provide benefits specified by law, with that insurance being voluntary. The general principle was that workers be able to get medical treatment and compensation regardless of whether the cause was the fault of the employer or the employee. In summary, "workers' compensation laws hold that industrial employers should assume costs of occupational disabilities without regard to any fault involved."[33] This removes employers from the liability of common law suits involving negligence.

In the "social fault doctrine," the employer is in the best position to prevent accidents and disease and therefore must be given incentive to do so. As the original system was very cumbersome, a series of safety codes gradually developed in the 19th and early 20th century specifying the employers' responsibility to provide safe working conditions. In the course of time, this ultimately led to the modern workers' compensation system.[11] The cost of workers' compensation has become part of the overhead of all industrial and manufacturing activity and is thus part of the cost of the product.

COMMON PRINCIPLES OF JUSTICE

"It is a general principle of common law litigation that a burden of proof lies upon the claimant (the 'plantiff')."[14] In systems in which employers' liability has existed or exists, the claimant must sue in an adversarial climate. The change to current workers' compensation systems of social insurance removes the burden of proof from the worker. The onus lies with the administering agency, such as a workers' compensation board, or the employer or an insurance company.

Whichever system is used, the evidence must be evaluated in the light of all the information obtainable so that there is a just outcome. Whether it be with judges in courts of law such as in the United States, with tribunals, or with compensation boards as exist in Canada, the standard of proof is that prescribed by law in the setting of a law court. Medical opinion is part of the evidence, but the final outcome is based on administrative or legal decisions. In practice, as each agency usually receives a large number of applications on a daily basis, each application must be dispatched in a timely manner. Because absolute proof may be lacking at a particular time, the final decision is often a balance of probabilities. The decision is found in favor of the claimant when the issue remains in doubt.

Various terms are used to describe work-related disease. The old term "industrial" is commonly understood to be equivalent to work-related disease but may be confusing, as it can apply only to scheduled disorders in some jurisdictions. A similar objection can be raised to the term "occupational disease," because specific occupations may not be covered by the legislation. These terms are still used commonly but will likely be replaced by "work-related" disease as the legislation becomes modified. The disease may be one caused exclusively by occupational exposure, or, if it occurs among the population at large in the particular circumstance, then work exposure might be a significant contributing cause. Disease is equated to accident in Ontario legislation for the management of compensation.[29] Such designation also exists in other jurisdictions.

As there is often uncertainty because of lack of knowledge or information concerning hazards and exposure, there is much latitude allowed in determination. Laskin draws attention to the nine guidelines set forward by Sir Bradford Hill in 1965, which are widely used.[18] They are strength, consistency, specificity and temporality of the association, biological gradients, plausibility, coherence, experiment, and analogy. These are quoted here to indicate the analysis to which evidence may be subjected. Work need not be the sole cause of a disease for disability to be compensable.[19] If work circumstances seem to have contributed to the disorder in a balance of probabilities, then the worker can be compensated in British and Canadian case law.

CURRENT WORKERS' COMPENSATION MANAGEMENT

Although the basic intent of workers' compensation is to provide compensation for work-related injury and disease, it does not cover all worker health problems. The statutes generally state that benefits are given for "personal injury caused by accidents arising out of and in the course of employment."[33] The interpretation of this is not uniform. Various states and provinces have their own lists of recognized occupational disease and coverage (see Chart IV[33] for details).

Compensation laws in the United States are elective or compulsory.[33] Under elective law, the employer may accept or reject coverage. If the law is rejected, then the major benefits of the law dealing with the rights of suit are lost to the employer. The workers' compensation legislation is compulsory throughout the United States and Canada with the exception of New Jersey, South Carolina, and Texas in the United States.

Employers are generally protected from damage suits for work-related injuries and diseases. Theoretically, if an employee rejects or is allowed to reject workers' compensation and sues the employer, then the three common law defenses of the assumption of risk, the negligence of fellow employees, and contributory negligence can be used by the employer.

RIGHTS AND DUTIES VERSUS DISCRETIONARY POWERS

Workers' compensation legislation in Canada creates rights and duties of the administering body but also creates a range of discretionary powers.[15] These rights and duties are laid down as a matter of law in the legislation governing the creation of the administering body. For example, a claim for a prescribed industrial disease must be considered if it is defined in the legislation. However, the administering body may have discretion as to the amount it awards or whether rehabilitation is offered.

The wide spectrum of varying legislation within each U.S. state and Canadian province indicates that administering bodies must be responsive to the marketplace of the area they serve. There is heterogeneity of industry, political climate, economy, geographic factors, and stakeholder attitudes in each regional area. Government agencies provide legislative guidelines and watchdog functions. It is not surprising that there is constant ongoing change within that environment. For example, in the United States, in 1972, a national commission found that state laws were not living up to their potential. The commission made 84 recommendations for improvement, of which 19 were termed essential. In 1976, another national policy group made further recommendations. A permanent federal body was established in the U.S. Department of Labor to oversee the work of state compensation programs. Arising from this have been increased growth and development in state compensation laws. These have assumed a more prominent role in the social insurance system of the United States. Task forces have rejected attempts to replace the state programs with a unified federal program. Occasional attempts that have been made to give the federal government a direct role through legislation introduced to Congress have always been unsupported. Workers' compensation acts in Canada were enacted under the purview of the provinces. Twelve autonomous boards and commissions exist, with each jurisdictional government's being responsible to the laws. This system differs from that in the United States, where the bulk of workers' compensation is administered through private insurance companies.

The common objectives underlying the compensation laws may be summarized as follows.

1. The laws provide prompt and reasonable income benefits as well as medical benefits for workers who have been subject to work accidents, regardless of fault. This includes income benefits for their dependents.

2. The laws provide a single remedy rather than the costly, time-consuming legal action that arises out of personal injury litigation. There are no legal or witness costs.

3. The law removes the necessity for dependence on public and private fund sources that might occur in uncompensated work accident or disease.

4. The law encourages employers to have appropriate interest in safety, accident prevention, and rehabilitation through experience rating.

5. The law promotes the objective study of the cause of accidents and hazards without punitive intent, with the aim of reducing these events and the concomitant suffering.[33]

CURRENT PLANS

Each state has its own legislation, which has tended to reflect the political climate of that state.[16,30,31] Any skin disease believed to have arisen from the work of the individual can be accepted, as doubt is given "in favor of the worker."[16] The federally funded National Institute of Occupational Health and Safety is a resource for information and research.

The Federal Employees' Compensation Act (FECA), which provides compensation for federal government employees, and the Longshore and Harbor Workers' Compensation Act are excluded.

Six states and two territories of the United States and all the provinces of Canada require employers to insure in a state or provincial fund that has a monopoly on that insurance. Thirteen states allow competition either as a state fund or by private insurers. Occasionally, employers may be allowed to be self-insurers. This usually applies to large corporations that can therefore avoid the administrative costs associated with insurance policies. Twenty-eight states and the Longshore Act authorize group insurance for smaller employers, who pool their risks and liabilities. In 1988, this represented 14.8% of the total coverage pool. Self-insurance is permitted in 47 U.S. states. The Canadian trend has been to do away with self-insurance, which is generally restricted to interprovincial transportation, communications, Crown or statutory corporations, and provincial and municipal governments. Self-insurers may set up reserve funds if it were advantageous in terms of tax benefits.

COVERAGE

United States

Virtually all industrial employment is covered (see Chart II[33]). There may be a limit to the minimum number of workers employed, and certain specified employments may be excluded. For example, farm workers, domestic workers, and casual employees are usually excluded. Most legislations allow an option for those not covered to be covered on a voluntary basis. Major industries with interstate or interprovincial activities such as rail and merchant marine workers are excluded, having in place their own legislation.

Canada

Canadian federal law legislates matters of interprovincial health and safety regarding workers and provides guidelines for the enactment of provincial legislation.[25]

Each of the twelve Canadian jurisdictions has a Workers' Compensation Board of Commission (WCB).[4,5] These boards receive, process, and fund workers' claims. The funds to carry out the programs are raised from employers, who are assessed annually and to many of whom an experience rating scale applies. The Federal Merchant Seamen's Compensation Act and Government Employees' Compensation Act (GECA) are among the exclusions. There is an administrative arrangement between WCBs and the federal government whereby GECA claims are dealt with by provincial boards. Alberta's WCB handles GECA claims on behalf of the Yukon and Northwest territories.

Workers have the responsibility to ensure that a problem is reported as soon as possible. The report may be made by the worker, by a physician, by a person or organization acting on the worker's behalf, or by the employer. The worker has freedom of choice of physician. Some jurisdictions allow nonmedical equivalents of physicians. Workers' clinics under the sponsorship of unions have been established in a few areas.

Other Countries

Legislation differs widely from country to country.[25] In the United Kingdom, employers pay into the Industrial Injuries Scheme, and workers also contribute until their retirement. The work injury benefits are part of the national security system of that country. Industrial diseases are tabulated in schedules due to cause. Doctors determine if the applicant is suffering from a defined illness, they determine the extent of the disability, and they estimate how long it will last. A percentage rating is then made. The award that is decided on the basis of medical recommendation is purely an impairment award and is independent of other losses of earnings, which are covered by other parts of the British National Insurance program.

In Australia, each state and territory has its own workers' compensation legislation. Recently, there has been a move away from common law rights, because claims have risen alarmingly. Part of that rise was in the form of high litigation costs. With the move to compensation boards, there has been increased emphasis on prevention and rehabilitation. Reduplication of benefits from other sources of welfare legislation has been eliminated and costs have fallen remarkably.

New Zealand has had a far-reaching no-fault scheme with very broad coverage since 1974.[7] It covered the population for all types of accidents and has been funded by road users and employers. Although the total and administrative costs for the scheme have been among the lowest in the world, growing discontent from the source of funding and the election of a more right-wing government have seen the introduction of new legislation similar to that of other countries.[22]

In contrast to many countries, France has national coverage in the framework of its Social Security Code. Legislation is drafted at the national government level. A national sickness insurance fund provides benefits for various regions of the country and also provides funds for research.

OPERATING PRINCIPLES

The structure of compensation boards is generally similar. An administrative division is responsible for the maintenance of the physical and support structure. A financial services division is responsible for all financial matters. Assessments and collection departments oversee the collection of revenues in the amounts the employers are assessed.

Claims or client service departments are the entry point into the system for the reporting of work injuries and diseases. The claims officers are laypersons who are trained adjudicators in the workers' compensation system. They decide which claims can be settled immediately, the length of time funded off work, which cases should be referred to the rehabilitation department, and which cases should be referred to the board medical officers.

Rehabilitation departments help workers to return to productive activity by assessment of their potential and referral to the rehabilitative agency. The rehabilitation is often provided by an outside agency, but some larger operations have their own rehabilitation services.[25]

The medical department advises on medical aspects of claims adjudication and advises management on matters of medical policy. Some departments promote research. Clients with occupational disease, as opposed to "accident," are usually referred automatically to the medical department. The volume of this work has led to board medical officers not only providing medical input but in actual fact being the adjudicators.[14]

APPEAL

Workers have the right to appeal in matters of dispute. This is generally at two levels. The first is internal appeal, which is rapid, economic, and effective. Most organizations have an internal structure of one or more levels of senior experience to which appeal is made. Outside this informal internal structure lies external appeal.

There are three methods by which appeals may be heard in the United States. The first is the common law system, which is court based. Since most jurisdictions have dispensed with the right to sue, the trial court initially reviews a statutorily imposed agreement that the worker for his or her part and the employer or employer's insurer must have signed. If this agreement is judged fair by the court and settlement is made, then that is the end of the matter. In cases of continuing dispute, the matter may go to trial court, to a higher circuit court, and finally to the state supreme court. Lawyers may get a contingency fee in this circumstance.[16]

Most Canadian jurisdictions have an established administrative system. If an appeal has worked its way through the various internal levels of appeal, there is an arm's-length tribunal available. This is a quasi-legal system separate from outside the legislated workers' compensation authority, which is semijudicial but which functions in a nonadversarial climate. Some systems fund legal counsel for clients, and others allow unfunded advisers to assist workers in the preparation of their case. The final level of appeal is usually binding, with challenges of process being allowed to go to courts of law. In some jurisdictions, a final level of appeal lies within the board or commission.

A more isolated appeal system exists, termed the Combination System in the United States. It is semijudicial, and although it is more informal than the court system, it has many of the time-consuming encumbrances of the court system. Most legislations define a time after which final decisions are binding.

OCCUPATIONAL DISEASE

Occupational disease must arise out of and in the course of the employment or be peculiar to or characteristic of industrial processes. What is not covered is "ordinary disease of life."[33] There have been some attempts in some countries to offer universal coverage to workers when there has been an extensive social security net in place in those countries. This has usually been unsuccessful, however, because of the cost. The coverages are summarized in Chart IV.[33] The compensation is similar to that for injury, but some states do not provide permanent partial disability payments. As knowledge increases regarding the causes and natural histories of occupational diseases, the legislation and the coverage become amended. In addition, there is increasing recognition of the extended latent period of certain diseases, and allowance is being made for this by way of extension of the claim period.[27]

PREVENTION

Prevention services including safety engineering are usually provided within workers' compensation programs. In some Canadian provinces, this is provided separately by the provincial Departments of Labour. The incentive to good safety records lies in experience rating. A company's records are generally assessed annually by a rate-making service, which reports back to the insurer, whether state or private. The insurance body sets the rate for the coming year for that particular industry based on that information.[6]

REHABILITATION

Rehabilitation services may be provided within a commission or WCB or may be contracted out.[25] The cost of early consideration for rehabilitation may be financially beneficial.[26,32] The attending physician can suggest this if it is doubtful that recovery will ever be complete enough for the former occupation to be resumed.

PHYSICIAN'S ROLE

The responsibility of the attending practitioner in Canada and many U.S. jurisdictions is to report findings and opinion to the board or commission. Reports after periodic examinations are also necessary. There is the right to consultation, for other opinions, if there is reasonable request on the part of the worker, for medical need, or if the insurer feels there has been inadequate progress. The insurer is obliged to pay for the medical attendance.

The standard principles of occupational dermatology practice should be followed.[1,12,20] Opinion should be supported by current standards of investigation, including appropriate patch testing and use of material safety data sheets. If a site visit is required, approval of the insuring body should be obtained beforehand.[28]

Writing the Report

A report is always required by the workers' compensation authority and will often be requested by lawyers or workers' representatives. The patient's physician takes the role of a neutral, objective, and scientific observer in making the report. It is a disservice to the patient, to society, and to the demands of ethical medical practice to do otherwise. A different situation exists when the dermatologist is called as an expert witness by lawyers representing a plaintiff or defendant in an appeal or, in some jurisdictions, a law court. In that circumstance, the evidence is reviewed critically in the light of the interests of the lawyers representing their client. The expert witness gives opinion confined to the questions posed.

A useful guide to the completion of a report for dermatological cases is found in the American Medical Association (AMA) guidelines.[2] Reports should be objective and written concisely. Any opinion given should be supported by factual statement about the observations. If evaluation of the extent of impairment is requested, it should be given. There should be no estimate of disability. As suggested earlier, recommendation for early rehabilitation can be made if the examiner believes it would be cost-effective judged by the long-term outlook.

An objective written report written in a clear and concise style with a minimum number of confusing technical terms gives credibility and confidence to employers, the compensation system, and the client (the patient). Easily available references can be quoted to support a point made. It should be remembered that reports will be read initially by claims officers, who are laypersons and who process the majority of claims. As indicated earlier, most claims for occupational disease are passed on to medical officers and might be used later in the appeal process. The style of the report should accommodate all these interests. A guide to such reporting and certain useful definitions can be found in Appendices A and B of the AMA guidelines.[2]

Assessment of Impairment

The most common evaluation of patients with work-related disease is to determine the amount of *impairment* of function that the disorder has caused. This is the responsibility of the physician. The alteration in health status must be contrasted with the patient's *disability,* "which is an alteration of the patient's capacity to meet personal, social, or occupational demands, or to meet statutory or regulatory requirements." This is assessed by nonmedical means. The assessment is most commonly performed by an experienced official for the commission, the WCB, or the insurance company. The existence of an impairment does not necessarily imply a disability. Disability results only when an individual is unable to meet the functional obligations of his or her work.

Evaluation of impairment is a stepwise process. The patient's current clinical status is evaluated by the standard processes of history taking, physical examination, and relevant investigations. The findings are then analyzed to determine the nature and extent of loss of function. The next step is to compare the findings with the rating scale used by the insuring authority.[2] The final step consists of evaluation of the whole person as far as impairment goes.

No impairment is considered permanent until the condition is static or well stabilized or until maximum benefit of rehabilitation effort is seen.

Some systems, but not all, work under an apportionment principle by which awards are given as a percentage of the judged disability.

Disabilities are classified as either temporary or permanent and as either partial or total. Temporary partial disability exists when a worker can still work at some job during the recovery period. Compensation would therefore represent the difference between wages before the injury and those earned during the period of injury. This situation is less common than that of temporary total disability. In the latter condition, the worker cannot work but is expected to be able to return to work within a defined period of time. There is commonly, but not always, a waiting period before benefits are paid in the United States. In Canada, benefits are generally payable the day after injury. Payments are usually based on a worker's average earnings but with a maximum and a minimum. Each jurisdiction has its own regulations, which should be consulted.

Permanent partial disability exists when the impairment results in permanent inability to compete in industry. Benefits are provided as compensation for the loss of future earnings. This may be managed in one of two ways: When a scheduled injury is defined in the regulations, the amount and conditions are fixed by legislation. This would apply whether or not the worker were working. The benefits are for a specified period of time the length of which depends on the part of the body that is injured. The other method of payment is nonscheduled. The compensation is a percentage of the difference between the wage earnings before and after the disablement.

The worker who is determined to be permanently and totally disabled is one who is judged never able to work again and for whom medical treatment or rehabilitation effort gives no promise of that. The amounts paid vary from jurisdiction to jurisdiction but are generally two-thirds of average wages with some addition for dependents in the United States. In Canada, generally, 75% of gross or 90% of net earnings are awarded. Some jurisdictions pay the benefit for a defined period of time. Others give it for life. There are defined maximums and minimums.

In situations in which the payment is relatively small, lump-sum settlements are made so as to reduce the cost of administration for the payment of benefits over a long period.

Fitness for Work

The physician's opinion on a worker's fitness for work is based on knowledge of the patient's current functional state and an understanding of the physical and mental demands of the patient's work. A site visit or inquiry of the employer may be necessary before that opinion can be given. Most commonly, a detailed discussion with the patient revealing the patient's day-to-day occupational activities provides enough information to produce that opinion.

Litigation

Physicians may be required to appear in an appeal or in a law court in some jurisdictions. As in all medicolegal situations, the role of the witness should be clarified beforehand. It should include a statement of responsibility for remuneration of these services if that is not in documented form at the time of request.

The clinician may be a witness if called as the client's specialized attendant. He or she may be an expert witness called at the request of the appeal tribunal or representatives of either side. In this circumstance there should be full clarification of the role. A written expert report may be required beforehand.

Again, neutral objectivity is expected of the physician whether called on behalf of the worker, on behalf of the insuring body, or as an expert witness.

In court or tribunal appearances, the general advice on deportment and preparation for the hearing as suggested in medicolegal texts should be followed. Reference texts or photocopies of references likely to be used should be brought to the hearing. Appearance by a physician at an appeal hearing is much more prevalent in the United States. In Canada, provision of written expert opinion or evidence is sufficient in the majority of cases.

CURRENT PROBLEMS

Rising costs are a problem. In 1991, the cost of workers' compensation in the United States had doubled during the previous five years.[33] This represented a 50% increase in the $42.9 billion spent by employers on insurance or self-insurance against work-related injuries. In 39 states, there is now an annual adjustment based on the state average weekly wage. For an idea of the extent of coverage, in 1988, 87% of all wage and salary employees in the United States were covered by work injury laws. This meant 91.3 million workers with a payroll of $2 trillion (84% of all civilian wage and salary payments).

The Canadian situation is similar. About 60% of the workforce (approximately 10.9 million workers) is covered under worker's compensation. Benefits paid out in 1991 were close to C$7 billion. Assessment revenues for the estimated 640,000 employer accounts totaled C$5.3 billion (Assocation of Workers' Compensation Boards of Canada source).

Cost containment is an issue that concerns the whole of industry. Cost containment concerns the regulations that provide "for a more efficient and equitable workers' compensation system that reduces claim costs while providing adequate benefits to workers and controls costs to employers." Employers, unions, individual workers, and insuring bodies are all equally affected. Consequently there is much continuing joint activity. The various U.S. strategies to reduce medical costs have been summarized recently.[23,34]

BASIS OF BENEFITS

In Canada, there is a movement away from the so-called "meat chart" in which benefits are paid on the basis of a clinical ratings schedule. The tendency is toward payment based on wage loss. Permanent disability awards are usually classified as scheduled and nonscheduled in the United States, with heavy reliance on the AMA guidelines for determination of amount.[2]

LIABILITY

Although there is reasonable concern that work-related skin conditions are underdiagnosed, there is also evidence of possible overdiagnosis. A critical study of 250 workers from a background of 14 different industries showed that only 127 (51%) had skin findings consistent with workplace exposure.[24] Although those patients also had more socioeconomic stress factors than normal, this study raises concern that strict criteria be applied to the diagnosis.

In summary, workers' compensation legislation is a mosaic of different schemes from country to country, province to province, and state to state. Despite the fact that those differences represent the individual character of each area, there is still a common theme—the theme of social welfare legislation that attempts to carry a public no-fault responsibility as part of daily work-related activity.

REFERENCES

1. Adams RM (ed): Occupational Skin Disease, 2nd ed. Philadelphia, W.B. Saunders, 1990.
2. American Medical Association: Guides to the Evaluation of Permanent Impairment, 3rd ed. Chicago, American Medical Association, 1989.
3. Annual Supplement to 1992 Analysis of Workers' Compensation Laws. U.S. Chamber Publication #0295. Washington, DC, U.S. Chamber of Commerce, 1992.
4. Association of Workers' Compensation Boards of Canada: Benefit Comparisons as of January 1, 1992. Edmonton, Alberta, 1992.
5. Association of Workers' Compensation Boards of Canada: Comparison of Workers' Compensation Legislation in Canada. Edmonton, Alberta, 1991.
6. Association of Workers' Compensation Boards of Canada: Workers' Compensation Experience Rating Programs in Canada. Edmonton, Alberta, 1991.
7. Coney S: New Zealand: Accident compensation changes. Lancet 338:1583–1584, 1991.
8. Encyclopedia Britannica Macropedia. Chicago, Encyclopedia Britannica, 15th ed, vol 18, 1974, p 523.
9. Encyclopedia Britannica Micropedia. Chicago, Encyclopedia Britannica, 15th ed, vol 10, 1974, p 749.
10. Encyclopedia Britannica Macropedia. Chicago, Encyclopedia Britannica, 15th ed, vol 9, 1974, p 528.
11. Encyclopedia Britannica Macropedia. Chicago, Encyclopedia Britannica, 15th ed, vol 8, 1974, pp 696–698.
12. Hindson C: Investigation of industrial dermatitis. In Griffiths WAD, Wilkinson DS (eds): Essentials of Industrial Dermatology. Oxford, Blackwell Scientific Publications, 1985, pp 24–37.
13. Hunter D: The Diseases of Occupation, 6th ed. London, Hodder & Stoughton, 1978, pp 744–790.
14. Ison TG: Compensation for Industrial Disease under the Workers' Compensation Act of Ontario. Toronto, Industrial Disease Standards Panel, 1989, p 4.
15. Ison TG: Compensation for Industrial Disease under the Workers' Compensation Act of Ontario. Toronto, Industrial Disease Standards Panel, 1989, p 3.
16. Ladou J: Workers' compensation. In Adams RM (ed): Occupational Skin Disease, 2nd ed. Philadelphia, W.B. Saunders, 1990, pp 280–288.
17. Larson A: Workers' compensation reform: The Canadian example. In Proceedings of the Annual Convention of the Association of Workers' Compensation Boards of Canada. Yellowknife, NYT, 1987, pp 20–27.
18. Laskin JI: Commentary on Ison TG: Compensation for Industrial Disease under the Workers' Compensation Act of Ontario. Toronto, Industrial Disease Standards Panel, 1989, p 49.
19. Lippel K: Commentary on Ison TG: Compensation for Industrial Disease under the Workers' Compensation Act of Ontario. Toronto, Industrial Disease Standards Panel, 1989, pp 58–59.
20. Maibach HI (ed): Occupational and Industrial Dermatology, 2nd ed. Chicago, Year Book, 1987.
21. Mathias CGT: The cost of occupational skin disease. Arch Dermatol 121:332–334, 1985.
22. Morel V: Personal communication.
23. National Council on Compensation Insurance: Cost Containment and Reform Activity Report, vol 1, 1991, pp 1–5.
24. Plotnick H: Analysis of 250 consecutively evaluated cases of workers' disability claims for dermatitis. Arch Dermatol 126:782–786, 1990.
25. Ross JB: The administration of workers' compensation in Canada. Int J Dermatol 29:548–552, 1990.
26. Ross JB: The extended patient: Occupational dermatology and the Canadian dermatologist. Can J Dermatol 1:36–39, 1989.
27. Ross JB: Prevention of occupational disease: Problems of data collection for adequate surveillance. Can Med Assoc J 147:1443–1445, 1992.

28. Rycroft RJG: Occupational site survey: Principles and significance. In Maibach HI (ed): Occupational and Industrial Dermatology, 2nd ed. Chicago, Year Book, 1987, pp 3–5.
29. Starkman DKL: Commentary on Ison TG: Compensation for Industrial Disease under the Workers' Compensation Act of Ontario. Toronto, Industrial Disease Standards Panel, 1989, p 66.
30. State Workers' Compensation Administration Profiles. U.S. Department of Labor, Washington, DC, 1991.
31. State Workers' Compensation Laws. U.S. Department of Labor, Washington, DC, 1992.
32. Strautins P, Hall W: Does early referral to an on-site rehabilitation program predict an early return to work? J Occup Health Safety (Aust) 5:137–143, 1989.
33. U.S. Chamber of Commerce: Analysis of Workers' Compensation Laws. Washington, DC, 1992, p vii.
34. Workers' Compensation Research Institute: Medical cost containment in workers' compensation. In WRCI Research Brief, vol 6. Cambridge, MA, 1990, pp 1–7.

RONALD GOLDNER, MD, FACP

WORK-RELATED IRRITANT CONTACT DERMATITIS

Clinical Associate Professor
Department of Dermatology
University of Maryland School of Medicine
Baltimore, Maryland

Reprint requests to:
Ronald Goldner, MD
1101 Saint Paul Street, Suite 410
Baltimore, MD 21202

It is well recognized that irritant contact dermatitis is the most frequent cause of occupational skin disease.[13] Irritation is best defined as a toxic reaction to chemicals or other environmental insults, and irritant contact dermatitis is defined as a condition caused by direct chemical injury to the skin but that does not involve sensitization. Approximately 75% of occupational contact dermatitis is nonimmunologic in nature.[10,13]

Despite numerous protective mechanisms, the skin remains vulnerable to new irritants found in the workplace. Since there is no reliable confirmatory test for irritation, the diagnosis depends on an accurate history in terms of exposure to the suspected irritant that is consistent with the clinical appearance, distribution, and course of the eruption.[20] Patch testing should always be performed to confirm the absence of allergic contact dermatitis.[8]

Predisposing factors for occupational skin disease usually take on a secondary role when occupational physicians are confronted with a patient claiming a work-related skin condition. Certain factors related to the workplace and certain factors intrinsic to the worker must be combined to confirm the diagnosis of a work-related skin disorder. Shmunes has categorized the job-related predisposing factors for occupational dermatoses as seen in Table 1.[24] Host-related factors, on the other hand, are those that represent variations within normal that predispose to work-related skin disease (Table 2).[24]

The types of irritation seen in the workplace have been classified into eight distinct types as

TABLE 1. Job-related Factors for Occupational Dermatoses

Amount of wet work performed
Number of irritating chemicals contacted
Exposure to heat, cold, humidity, vibration, or radiation
Biologic agent exposure
Trauma

seen in Table 3.[2,10] The most common occupational irritants include water, skin cleansers, industrial cleansing agents, alkalis, acids, oils, organic solvents, oxidizing agents, reducing agents, plants, and animal products.[3,21] Strong irritants within any occupation are easily recognized because they cause rapid injury to the skin that is manifested by burning and inflammation. Adams includes wet cement, fibrous glass, ethylene oxide, and hydrofluoric acid as common examples of strong occupational irritants.[1] Most irritants, like contact sensitizers, have a molecular weight of less than 1,000. Because penetration of a compound decreases with increasing molecular weight, therefore the solubility, the pH, and the presence of reactive groups also contribute to a compound's irritating potential.[3]

COMMON IRRITANTS

In order to better understand work-related dermatitis, we must examine the previously mentioned irritants in more detail.

Water

Many occupations include some form of wet work. Prolonged contact with water can cause dry skin by dissolving the hygroscopic substances on the surface that are needed to keep the skin pliable. This is facilitated by prior removal of the surface lipid layer. Various elements in hard water can deposit into skin fissures, causing mechanical irritation.[3,21]

Skin Cleansers

Most detergents, soaps, and waterless cleansers containing organic solvents can irritate the skin. Usually they raise the pH and dissolve lipids on the surface, but added abrasives such as silica and sand cause further mechanical damage.[3]

Industrial Cleansing Agents

Industrial-strength cleansing products can be used for domestic as well as industrial cleaning and include detergents, surfactants, wetting agents, and emulsifiers. The irritating effect of each is of course different depending on the chemistry of the agent. Most have an alkaline pH, but, even when neutral, they can remove the surface lipid film from the stratum corneum. Proteins can thus be denatured and cell membranes damaged so as to further add to the irritation.[21]

TABLE 2. Host-related Predisposing Factors

Dry skin
Genetic background (fair skin)
Aging skin
Hairiness
Sweating

TABLE 3. Types of Irritation

Acute irritant dermatitis
Irritant reaction
Delayed acute irritant dermatitis
Cumulative irritant contact dermatitis
Traumatic irritant dermatitis
Pustular and acneiform dermatitis
Nonerythematous irritation
Friction irritation

Alkalis

Alkaline solutions such as soap, ammonia, sodium hydroxide, potassium hydroxide, cement, lime, sodium silicate, trisodium phosphate, and amines, including epoxy hardeners, are present in various industries. Irritant dermatitis can result from alkali saponification of skin surface lipids within many of those industries.[21]

Acids

Sulfuric, hydrochloric, nitric, chromic, and hydrofluoric acids are the most common industrial inorganic acids, whereas acetic and oxalic acids are the most often used organic acids. Hydrochloric acid is used by masons for cleaning bricks and stones. Chromic acid can be used for rustproofing iron, and hydrofluoric acid is used for etching glass.[3,17,23]

Oils

Metalworkers use cutting oils as coolants that usually contain oil, water, an emulsifier, an antioxidant, an anticorrosive agent, and a preservative. These oils, when mixed with particles of metal, stick to the skin surface, causing further irritation. The worker often complicates the problem by attempting to remove the residue with harmful organic solvents.[21]

Organic Solvents

Almost all organic solvents serve as irritants usually by dissolving surface lipids and cell membrane lipids. Solvents are widely used to clean textiles and metals and are also an important part of the graphics, painting, and wood-finishing industries. Most contain benzene, toluene, and aromatic petroleum as well as alcohols. Diesel oil, fuel oil, and thinner are prime examples of the irritating solvents used by workers.[3,21]

Oxidizing Agents

Oxidants, such as benzoyl peroxide and cyclohexanone peroxide, are used to harden polyester resins in the plastics industry. Some are also used in hair bleaching and for bleaching textiles, oils, and flour. Sodium hypochlorite is often used by printers and dye workers to clean their hands.[3,21]

Reducing Agents

Phenols, hydrazines, and thioglycolates are reducing agents often found in the workplace. Hairdressers can use either alkaline ammonium thioglycolate or acid glyceryl monothioglycolate to alter the curve of hair by breaking the disulfide bonds within hair keratin.[3,21]

Plants

Plant components often act as irritants. The most common are citrus peel, flower bulbs, garlic, spices, onion, cucumber, asparagus, mustard, barley, corn, and buttercup. It must also be appreciated that primary irritation and foreign body granulomas can result from penetration of the skin by twigs or trichromes of the plant.[6]

Animal Products

Caterpillars, carpet beetles, and moths can cause a vesicular or papular irritant dermatitis. Wet work with meat, fish, and shellfish can also be responsible for irritant reactions in restaurant workers or those in the canning industry.[21]

IRRITANTS IN COMMON OCCUPATIONS

Mathias and Morrison in 1988 reviewed the results of the U.S. Bureau of Labor Statistics Annual Survey of Occupational Injuries and Illness from 1973 through 1984.[15] Agricultural and manufacturing occupations have consistently had the highest rates and numbers of cases, respectively, but 40% of all occupational illness was shown to be due to skin disease.[1,4,7,14]

Most investigators agree that cumulative irritant dermatitis is more common than the allergic type, but this could be responsible for the increased penetration of allergens with the development of superimposed allergic contact dermatitis. Patch testing is thus mandatory in all cases of suspected occupational contact dermatitis.[8,18] If we examine some common occupations more closely, we can better appreciate the irritants to which workers are exposed.[2,10,13]

Agriculture Workers

Even though the pattern of farming in the United States has changed from the small family farm to large corporate farming, the incidence of occupational skin disease has remained high. Pesticides, artificial fertilizers, disinfectants, cleansers, gasoline, diesel oil, plants and grains, and animal secretions are the source of most of the irritation.[1,11,20]

Automobile Workers

Mechanics obviously have the greatest exposure to automotive irritants. These include solvents, oils, paints, cleansers, gasoline, and diesel fuel. Body and fender workers also have exposure to abrasives and adhesives.[1,13,20]

Bakers

In general, bakers and pastry workers mix flour to form batter, dough, and various fillings. Such exposure produces skin irritation from wet dough, detergents, cleansers, acids, spices, essential oils, and fruit juices.[1,3,17]

Bartenders

Within this profession, various ingredients can be combined with alcohol or soda to form a cocktail or mixed drink. Wet-work dermatitis is thus very common due to bartenders' frequent exposure to water, alcohol, fruit juices, soaps, and detergents.[3,20]

Butchers

Most butchers are known to cut and trim meat, but they are also exposed to poultry, fish, and seafood. Butchers' potential skin irritants include water, cleansers, soaps, detergents, and spices, as well as meat, fish, and fowl entrails.[1,3,20]

Carpenters

Cabinetmakers and woodworkers construct and repair furniture and other wooden articles. Sawdust irritation is thus very common, but other skin irritants include stains, solvents, glues, abrasives, and wood preservatives.[1,3,20]

Dental Workers

Dentists, dental assistants, and dental hygienists all wear gloves during their workday. They examine, extract, fill, straighten, clean, and replace teeth within the oral cavity. The most common skin irritants they contact are soaps, abrasives, adhesives, plasters, germicidals, and solvents.[9,19]

Electricians

Electrical workers build and repair electric appliances, fixtures, and circuits. They may have irritating contact with resins, soldering flux, fiberglass, or solvents.[1,3]

Health Care Workers

This category includes physicians, nurses, pharmacists, podiatrists, lab technicians, and physician's assistants. As a whole, this group can be exposed to soaps, detergents, disinfectants, and medications. Ethylene oxide from sterilization is still a potential cutaneous hazard, and chlorhexidine scrub has produced a number of reports of irritant contact dermatitis.[9,19]

Jewelers

Most jewelers now clean or repair jewelry rather than manufacture it. The irritants that they are exposed to include metal cleansers, acids, alkalis, solvents, abrasives, adhesives, and soldering flux.[1,3,20]

Machinists

Occupations involving operation or repair of machinery include machine tool operator, lathe operator, shaper, grinder, and metalworker. Most of the dermatitis seen in this group arises from the irritating properties of soluble coolants and subsequent exposure to solvents and abrasive hand cleansers.[1,5,13]

Masons and Cement Workers

Cement finishers, pavers, and masons are all exposed to wet cement. The irritation seems to be related to the highly alkaline calcium hydroxide rather than to sensitization to chromium. The addition of sand and gravel to form concrete increases the irritant potential.[1,3,20]

Office Workers

This broad category comprises secretaries, typists, and computer operators. Irritant exposure includes using copy machines, carbonless copy paper, typewriters, and computers with visual display terminals, in addition to simply being in the office environment. The most common irritants are soaps, solvents, papers, inks, ammonia, and photocopy toners.[11,12,14]

Photographers

Those in this profession often develop their own photographs, which provides potential irritation from the developing solutions, reducers, and toning agents used. The most prevalent irritants are acids, solvents, oxidizing agents, and reducing agents.[11,14,20]

Printers

Modern printing methods utilize four basic techniques: letterpress, gravure, lithography (offset printing), and stencil (screen process). All use metal plates or cylinders in contact with various inks. Recently, however, a photosensitive printing process has become popular. Common skin irritants among printers are acids, alkalis, solvents, gum arabic, soaps, detergents, inks, and acrylates.[1,14,16]

Roofers

A roof may be either flat or pitched, but it is first covered with hot tar over an insulating material. Then it is often finished with tile, slate, asphalt, or wooden shingles. Thus tar, asphalt, solvents, putty, fiberglass, and hand cleansers cause abundant irritation.[1]

Tannery and Leather Workers

This industry involves considerable exposure to irritants because all hides removed from animals must be dried, preserved, cleaned, and, finally, tanned into leather. The potential irritants are acids, alkalis, lime, enzymes, solvents, cleansers, and ammonia.[1,11,13]

Textile Workers

The textile industry today is almost totally mechanized, but the actual materials or fibers utilized may be of animal or chemical origin. Exposure to acids, alkalis, lubricating oils, solvents, and bleaching agents can contribute to irritant dermatitis.[1,14,22]

APPROACH TO DIAGNOSIS

It is now obvious that irritant contact dermatitis in the workplace has become sufficiently common in the practices of occupational physicians. These physicians are aware of the need to examine the causal agents within an occupation as well as various secondary contributing factors. It is likewise important that the history and physical examination be thorough and complete in order to substantiate a diagnosis of work-related irritant contact dermatitis.

Often, a site visit to the workplace is necessary to better understand the exact nature of a patient's occupation. Patience and an investigative spirit are also required to systematically solve the problem of irritant dermatitis in the workplace. Logical time relationship between exposure and skin disease must be established, and an accurate description of occupational tasks should include (1) material and chemical exposure, (2) how the materials are handled, (3) the protective clothing worn, and (4) methods used for skin cleansing.

Patch testing is still an essential part of evaluating any patient for irritant contact dermatitis. Testing with unknown chemicals brought from the workplace must be done cautiously, because false-positive or false-negative reactions can occur. Material safety data sheets should be read on each suspected irritant, and a preliminary open test is often advisable.[8,18]

PREVENTION

The problems of irritant contact dermatitis in the workplace are best solved by prevention. A multidisciplinary approach is necessary to reduce exployees' exposure to irritants. Education of workers and supervisors goes a long way to decrease that potential exposure.

A comfortable work environment increases the resistance of the skin to irritants by regulation of the ventilation, temperature, and humidity within the workplace. Mechanical irritation from the grinding effect of particles can often be reduced by physical barriers. It is imperative that skin exposure to potential irritants be kept to a minimum. Gloves, protective clothing, and barrier creams can be used judiciously as the occupation permits. The preliminary identification of hazardous irritating materials, as well as high-risk employees, is helpful in preventing an "epidemic" of occupational irritant contact dermatitis.[4,7,11]

THERAPY AND PROGNOSIS

The treatment of irritant contact dermatitis of the workplace depends upon the stage of the irritation. The acute phase is best treated with astringent soaks, topical or systemic corticosteroids, and antihistamines. The chronic phase is managed by moisturizing the dry skin and healing the fissures with topical corticosteroid ointments. Antibiotics are of course used for secondary pyoderma.

When preventative and therapeutic measures fail, then skin impairment resulting in loss of time from work may develop. Rehabilitation efforts should be aimed at restoring the economic and vocational usefulness of the employee. If a change in job within the workplace is not possible, the worker may need to receive workers' compensation disability payments while considering retraining for a new occupation.[13,14]

Irritant contact dermatitis of the workplace does not appear randomly. It is the result of many predisposing factors in the environment as well as in the host. Once recognized, these factors can be isolated and hopefully reduced. Early job counseling will be extremely helpful to patients with high-risk skin diseases and can prevent later disappointment in the job market.[1,13,24]

REFERENCES

1. Adams RM: Occupational Skin Disease, 2nd ed. Philadelphia, W.B. Saunders, 1990, pp 578–691.
2. Bason M, Lammintausta K, Maibach HI: Irritant dermatitis. In Marzulli FN, Maibach HI (eds): Dermatotoxicology, 4th ed. New York, Hemisphere Publishing Corp, 1991, pp 223–253.
3. Bruze M, Emmett EA: Occupational exposures to irritants. In Jackson EM, Goldner R (eds): Irritant Contact Dermatitis. New York, Marcel Dekker, 1990, pp 81–106.
4. Cronin E: Contact Dermatitis. Edinburgh, Churchill-Livingstone, 1980.
5. de Boer EM, van Ketel WG, Bruynzeel DP: Dermatoses in metal workers. Contact Dermatitis 20:212–218, 1989.
6. Epstein WL: House and garden plants. In Jackson EM, Goldner R (eds): Irritant Contact Dermatitis. New York, Marcel Dekker, 1990, pp 127–165.
7. Fisher AA: Contact Dermatitis, 3rd ed. Philadelphia, Lea & Febiger, 1986.
8. Goldner R: Clinical tests. In Jackson EM, Goldner R (eds): Irritant Contact Dermatitis. New York, Marcel Dekker, 1990, pp 201–218.
9. Hogan DJ: Contact dermatitis in health care workers. In Exogenous Dermatoses: Environmental Dermatitis. Boca Raton, CRC Press, 1990.
10. Lammintausta K, Maibach HI: Contact dermatitis due to irritation. In Adams R (ed): Occupational Skin Disease, 2nd ed. Philadelphia, W.B. Saunders, 1990, pp 1–25.
11. Maibach HI, Gellin G: Occupational and Industrial Dermatology. Chicago, Year Book, 1982.
12. Marks JG: Dermatologic problems of office workers. Dermatol Clin 6:61–66, 1988.

13. Marks JG, DeLeo VA: Contact and Occupational Dermatology. St. Louis, Mosby–Year Book, 1992.
14. Mathias CGT: Occupational dermatoses. J Am Acad Dermatol 19:1107–1114, 1988.
15. Mathias CGT, Morrison JH: Occupational skin disease, United States. Arch Dermatol 124:1519–1524, 1988.
16. Nethercott JR: Dermatitis in the printing industry. Dermatol Clin 6:75–79, 1988.
17. Nethercott JR, Holness DL: Occupational dermatitis in food handlers and bakers. J Am Acad Dermatol 21:485–490, 1989.
18. Rietschel RL: Patch testing in occupational hand dermatitis. Dermatol Clin 6:43–46, 1988.
19. Rudzki E, Rebandel P, Grzywa Z: Patch tests with occupational contactants in nurses, doctors and dentists. Contact Dermatitis 20:247–250, 1989.
20. Rycroft RJG: Occupational dermatoses. In Champion RH, Burton JL, Ebling FJG (eds): Rook/Wilkinson/Ebling Textbook of Dermatology, 5th ed. Oxford, Blackwell, 1992, pp 763–776.
21. Rycroft RJG, Wilkinson JD: Irritants and sensitizers. In Champion RH, Burton JL, Ebling FJG (eds): Rook/Wilkinson/Ebling Textbook of Dermatology, 5th ed. Oxford, Blackwell, 1992, pp 717–754.
22. Sheretz EF: Contact dermatitis in textile industry workers. Am J Contact Dermatitis 2:69, 1991.
23. Shewmake SW, Anderson B: Hydrofluoric acid burns. Arch Dermatol 115:593–596, 1979.
24. Shmunes E: Predisposing factors in occupational skin disease. Dermatol Clin 6:7–13, 1988.
25. Shupack JL, Romano SJ: Human skin reactions to ethylene oxide. J Lab Clin Med 98:723, 1981.

D. LINN HOLNESS, MD

CHARACTERISTIC FEATURES OF OCCUPATIONAL DERMATITIS:

Epidemiologic Studies of Occupational Skin Disease Reported by Contact Dermatitis Clinics

From the Department of Occupational and Environmental Health
St. Michael's Hospital
University of Toronto

Reprint requests to:
D. Linn Holness, MD
Department of Occupational and Environmental Health
St. Michael's Hospital
30 Bond St.
Toronto, Ontario M5B 1W8
Canada

TYPE OF CONTACT DERMATITIS

Conventional wisdom says that greater than 70% of contact dermatitis is irritant in nature and that the remainder is allergic.[1] It is difficult to determine what the true percentage is, as most of the reported results relate to selected patient groups rather than the general population. Information regarding contact dermatitis is best obtained from large-scale epidemiological studies such as that of Meding and Swanbeck.[9] Their data suggest that irritant contact dermatitis (ICD) is more common but that there is variation depending on the exposures.

There is also variation in the reporting of the distribution of allergic contact dermatitis (ACD) and ICD in the selected populations of workers as reported by patch test centers. For instance, two groups of researchers have found a higher prevalence of ICD. Wall and Gebauer reported that ICD occurred in 71% of 993 workers with occupational skin disease, whom they assessed in Australia, while only 38% had ACD.[14] Goh and Soh reported a similar higher prevalence of ICD (66% ICD vs. 34% ACD) in Singapore.[4] Others have found a relatively equal distribution of ACD and ICD. These include values of 50% for ACD and 47% for ICD reported by Kanerva et al. in Finland,[6] 49% for ICD and 51% for ACD from Italy,[12] and 48% for ICD and 52% for ACD noted in Toronto.[5]

Fregert found a similarly equal representation of ICD and ACD in the female population he assessed in Sweden.[3] On the other hand, Fregert also noted more ACD among the male population (73% had ACD). The North American Contact Dermatitis Group (NACDG) also found a higher proportion with ACD (50% ACD vs. 30% ICD).[10] These differences may reflect different exposures and risks of sensitization and also differences in the age and sex distribution of the patients assessed.

AGE

There is relatively little information in the literature regarding age distribution of populations affected by occupationally related contact dermatitis. Wall and Gebauer noted 54% of the individuals they assessed with occupational skin disease were younger than 40.[14] Information from the NACDG found that those with occupationally related dermatitis were significantly younger than those with nonoccupational contact dermatitis.[10] Holness and Nethercott reported similar results.[5]

SEX

Most studies report the sex distribution of their population. Generally, men are overrepresented in occupationally related skin disease. This in part reflects the larger proportion of men in the workforce. However, even if this is taken into account, there still appears to be an overrepresentation of men. For example, in Fregert's population in Sweden, 66% were male.[3] Vestey et al. in Scotland reported that 46% of those with occupational dermatitis were male in comparison to 39% of all who were patch tested.[13] Of the Singapore population assessed by Goh and Soh, 71% were male.[4] Sertoli et al. noted that 34% of their entire patch test population were men; however, 45% of the patients with occupationally related problems were men.[12] The Australian experience of Wall and Gebauer found that 70% of those with occupational skin disease were male,[14] and Lachapelle and Tennstedt, in Belgium, found 56%.[8] The NACDG results indicate that 57% of those with occupationally related skin disease were male in comparison with only 42% with nonoccupationally related disease.[10] Similar numbers in the Toronto population were 69% and 40%, respectively.[5]

LOCATION OF DERMATITIS

There is relatively little information in the literature regarding the distribution of dermatitis among these populations. Often, only information related to the prevalence of hand dermatitis is noted. For example, Fregert noted that 94% of females and 84% of males had hand involvement.[3] Wilkinson et al. found that 69% had hand involvement and 23% arm involvement.[15] The North American experience and the experience specific to the Toronto clinic are reported in Table 1, again demonstrating that the majority had hand involvement.[5,10]

There has been even less information reported from the patch test clinic series regarding distribution of dermatitis related to diagnosis. Analysis of results from Toronto suggests that some locations are increased in both ACD and ICD and that others are preferentially represented in just one type.[5] Hand involvement is high in both occupational ACD and ICD, whereas involvement of the arms, face, and eyelids is increased in those with occupational ACD in comparison to those those with occupational ICD.

TABLE 1. Location of Dermatitis

	NACDG		Toronto	
	Occupational (N = 288)	Nonoccupational (N = 1,291)	Occupational (N = 801)	Nonoccupational (N = 816)
Location				
Hand	83	38	85	34
Arm	15	13	34	15
Leg	3	9	9	11
Foot	12	10	8	10
Face	11	23	9	25
Eyelids	1	6	4	17
Generalized	9	15	3	10
Trunk	4	10	5	12

NACDG = North American Contact Dermatitis Group.

LENGTH OF TIME WITH DERMATITIS

Several studies report some time factors. Wall and Gebauer noted that 57% of the patients they assessed with occupational skin disease had had their eruption for less than one year.[14] In Toronto, 61% of those with occupational dermatitis had had their problem for less than one year, whereas 51% of those with nonoccupational contact dermatitis had problems for less than one year.[5] The mean time of eruption prior to diagnosis in Toronto was 34 months for occupational and 49 months for nonoccupational contact dermatitis.[5] Those with occupational ICD had a shorter duration (28 months) compared to those with occupational ACD (37 months).[5]

PATCH TESTING

Many studies report the results of patch testing. Fewer have provided their results categorized by occupational and nonoccupational dermatitis (Table 2).[5,10,15] Such categorization provides an opportunity to compare the results and identify those allergens that are particularly related to occupational exposures. The allergens for which there appeared to be consistently increased positive results across the three studies were epoxy resin, mercapto mix, paraphenylenediamine, and potassium dichromate.

Some studies also report information about the results in males and females separately (Table 3).[5,8,15] There appears to be a consistent increase in positive responses to nickel sulphate in women and to potassium dichromate in men. Women tended to have more thiuram mix positives and men more black rubber mix positives.

Several studies report the results of patch test responses in the subgroup of the population that has had a diagnosis of occupational ACD (Table 4).[5,6,14] In this population there were increased positive responses to epoxy resin, paraphenylenediamine, thiuram mix, and potassium dichromate.

One can also compare the response to patch test allergens between those with occupational ACD and occupational ICD (Table 5).[5] Agents for which there was an odds ratio greater than two for the comparison of ACD to ICD included epoxy resin, thiuram mix, potassium dichromate, black rubber mix, carba mix,

TABLE 2. Patch Test Results—Comparison of Percentage of Positive Patch Test Results in Those with Occupational and Nonoccupational Contact Dermatitis

Author:	Nethercott		Holness		Wilkinson	
Location:	North Am		Toronto		England	
Years:	1987–1989		1980–1988		1970s	
Type of Dermatitis:	Nonocc	Occ	Nonocc	Occ	Nonocc	Occ
Number tested:	1,291	288	816	801	992	292
Substance						
Balsam of Peru	5.6	4.7	6.3	3.4	–	–
Benzyl peroxide	3.0	1.8	1.5	1.1	–	–
Black rubber mix/PPD mix	2.0	3.9	1.3	2.3	1.0	1.2
Carba mix	4.7	7.4	3.5	4.1	–	–
Cinnamic alcohol	5.3	5.0	6.6	3.5	–	–
Cinnamic aldehyde	4.2	3.9	4.0	3.9	–	–
Cobalt	–	–	5.7	9.8	4.1	2.7
Colophony	1.8	4.1	3.4	4.7	3.3	4.1
Diaminophenylmethane	2.6	2.8	2.0	3.3	–	–
Epoxy resin	2.3	4.6	1.1	6.4	1.5	4.1
Ethylenediamine	5.7	3.5	3.3	5.8	–	–
Formaldehyde	7.9	11.0	6.1	6.6	1.3	5.1
Fragrance mix	–	–	10.4	5.4	–	–
Mercapto mix	1.6	4.6	0.9	2.0	2.2	4.1
Mercaptobenzothiazole	1.7	5.1	0.9	1.8	–	–
Neomycin	7.6	5.0	4.6	3.0	–	–
Nickel	10.2	13.5	10.2	10.1	8.7	6.5
Paraphenylenediamine	5.5	10.3	4.5	8.5	2.3	4.1
Potassium dichromate	2.7	4.6	3.8	7.6	2.2	4.4
p-tert-butylphenol formaldehyde resin	2.0	1.1	0.9	1.6	–	–
Quaternium-15	6.9	8.8	2.6	2.9	–	–
Thiomersol	10.1	10.0	3.2	4.0	–	–
Thiuram mix	5.7	9.2	2.8	6.7	4.2	4.1
Woolwax alcohols	1.5	2.1	1.6	1.4	–	–

Nonocc = nonoccupational dermatitis; and Occ = occupational dermatitis.

mercaptobenzothiazole, balsam of Peru, fragrance mix, colophony, paraphenylenediamine, formaldehyde, cobalt, and mercapto mix.

FUTURE DIRECTIONS

Contact dermatitis clinics see a large number of individuals with occupationally related disease. Experience with those occupationally related cases has been reported by a variety of authors. In general, those with occupationally related dermatitis are more likely to be men and younger than those with nonoccupationally related contact dermatitis. With respect to distribution of dermatitis, the hands are

TABLE 3. Patch Test Results—Comparison of Percentage of Positive Patch Test Results in Those with Occupational and Nonoccupational Contact Dermatitis by Sex

Author:	Wilkinson		Holness		LaChapelle	
Location:	England		Toronto		Belgium	
Years:	1970s		1980–1988		(?) 1970s	
Sex:	Male	Female	Male	Female	Male	Female
Number tested:	232	60	573	281	225	175
Substance						
Balsam of Peru	–	–	3.9	2.8	5.8	8.6
Benzyl peroxide	–	–	0.3	2.6	–	–
Benzocaine	–	–	0.9	0.6	4.9	4.6
Black rubber mix/PPD mix	1.7	0	2.7	1.9	4.9	0.6
Carba mix	–	–	3.5	4.6	2.2	4.0
Cobalt	1.7	6	8.3	12.5	7.6	8.0
Colophony	4.7	1	3.3	7.5	2.2	2.3
Diaminophenylmethane	–	–	3.6	2.5	–	–
Epoxy resin	3.9	7	7.9	2.7	2.7	1.1
Ethylenediamine	–	–	6.3	4.2	0.9	1.7
Formaldehyde	5.2	5	5.2	10.0	2.7	5.1
Fragrance mix	–	–	6.3	7.1	–	–
Mercapto mix	3.9	5	2.4	0.7	1.8	1.7
Mercaptobenzothiazole	–	–	2.0	1.3	–	–
Neomycin	–	–	3.3	3.8	1.3	5.7
Nickel	3.2	15	5.1	20.6	4.0	20.6
Paraphenylenediamine	3.0	8	5.8	13.5	9.3	8.0
Potassium dichromate	5.6	0	8.4	5.3	17.3	9.7
p-tert-butylphenol formaldehyde resin	–	–	1.2	2.3	–	–
Thiuram mix	3.9	5	5.4	9.5	2.7	11.4
Woolwax alcohols (lanolin)	–	–	1.5	1.1	3.6	5.1

affected in the majority of cases. Occupational ACD tends to involve the arms, face, and eyelids more often than ICD.

The results of patch testing have been reported by a number of groups. They are somewhat difficult to compare, given the difference in populations from which the patients are drawn and equally the way in which the results are reported. In some cases, it is the entire population patch tested in the clinic; in other cases, all those with occupational skin disease; and in still others, more specifically only those with allergic occupational skin disease. Some groups also have reported results for both males and females. Even given these problems, there are still some clear trends as to which substances are overrepresented in workplace exposures. They tend to include potassium dichromate, epoxy resin, a variety of rubber products, and paraphenylenediamine.

Review of the literature related to the reporting of these results suggests that it would be most helpful if some uniformity of reporting of results were established so as to make comparison between groups easier. There is clearly some

TABLE 4. Patch Test Results—Percentage of Positive Patch Test Results in Those with Occupational Allergic Contact Dermatitis

Author:	Wall		Kanerva	Holness
Location:	Australia		Finland	Toronto
Years:	1980–1987		1974–1983	1980–1988
Sex:	Male	Female		
Number tested:	265	103	542	420
Substance				
Balsam of Peru	0.8	–	–	5.5
Benzyl peroxide	–	–	–	1.8
Benzocaine	–	–	–	0.8
Black rubber mix/PPD mix	2.0	1.0	–	4.0
Carba mix	–	1.0	–	6.9
Cobalt	11	5.7	3.0	14.2
Colophony	2.6	1.0	1.1	7.1
Diaminophenylmethane	–	–	–	4.0
Epoxy resin	9.5	2.0	13.1	11.7
Ethylenediamine	–	–	–	6.9
Formaldehyde	2.3	2.0	5.7	9.5
Fragrance mix	–	3.0	–	8.3
Mercapto mix	–	–	–	2.9
Mercaptobenzothiazole	5.3	2.0	–	3.2
Neomycin	–	–	0.2	2.7
Nickel	3	25	6.6	12.9
Paraphenylenediamine	1.5	9.6	–	13.5
Potassium dichromate	37	3.0	18.8	13.1
p-tert-butylphenol formaldehyde resin	2.0	3.0	1.0	2.0
Rubber materials	–	–	19.9	–
Thiuram mix	10	15	–	12.5
Woolwax alcohols (lanolin)	–	–	–	1.6

difference in the specific allergens that are used as part of a standard screening series in different jurisdictions; the concentration of the allergen employed also varies. However, as the information usually has been collected in a standardized manner in many settings, and is readily amenable to computerization, it should be relatively easy to generate basic descriptive information related to the population, or various subsets of the population. It would be through consistent reporting of such information that differences in responses to the various allergens might be noted between different populations. These differences could lead to hypothesis generation about both specific risk factors or various protective strategies that may vary between different jurisdictions and that could then be formally tested. This information could be of practical use to identify specific populations at risk and effective or ineffective strategies in reducing risk.

TABLE 5. Patch Test Results—Difference in Patch Test Results between Occupational Allergic and Irritant Contact Dermatitis, St. Michael's Hospital, 1980–1988

Substance	Irritant (N = 347)	Allergic (N = 378)	Odds Ratio*	p Value*
Balsam of Peru	1.3	5.3	5.0	0.005
Benzyl peroxide	0.5	1.4	2.0	0.562
Black rubber mix	0.6	4.2	8.6	0.005
Carba mix	1.2	6.9	5.7	0.002
Cobalt	5.7	14.0	2.5	0.007
Colophony	2.0	7.4	3.4	0.005
Diaminophenylmethane	2.8	2.8	0.9	0.823
Epoxy resin	0.9	12.5	20.7	0.000
Ethylenediamine	4.6	6.0	1.5	0.299
Formaldehyde	3.2	9.5	2.9	0.003
Fragrance mix	2.0	7.4	4.0	0.001
Mercapto mix	1.1	2.1	2.3	0.185
Mercaptobenzothiazole	0.5	2.4	5.3	0.136
Neomycin	3.4	3.0	0.9	0.797
Nickel sulphate	7.2	12.7	1.4	0.235
Paraphenylenediamine	3.7	13.7	3.4	0.000
p-tert-butylphenol formaldehyde resin	1.3	2.2	1.5	0.588
Potassium dichromate	1.7	13.5	10.4	0.000
Thiuram mix	0.6	12.2	20.7	0.000
Woolwax alcohols (lanolin)	1.2	1.2	0.9	0.923

* p values and odds ratios calculated by logistic regression analysis and corrected for age and sex.

REFERENCES

1. Adams RM: Allergic contact dermatitis. In Occupational Skin Disease, 2nd ed. Philadelphia, WB Saunders, 1990, p 26.
2. California Department of Industrial Relations. Occupational skin disease in California. January, 1992.
3. Fregert S: Occupational dermatitis in a 10-year material. Contact Dermatitis 1:96–107, 1975.
4. Goh CL, Soh SD: Occupational dermatoses in Singapore. Contact Dermatitis 11:288–293, 1984.
5. Holness DL, Nethercott JR: Comparison of occupational and non-occupational contact dermatitis, submitted for publication.
6. Kanerva L, Estlander T, Jolanki R: Occupational skin disease in Finland. Int Arch Occup Environ Health 60:89–94, 1988.
7. Keil JE, Shmunes E: The epidemiology of work-related skin disease in South Carolina. Arch Dermatol 119:650–654, 1983.
8. Lachapelle JM, Tennstedt D: Epidemiological survey of occupational contact dermatitis of the hands in Belgium. Contact Dermatitis 5:244–248, 1979.
9. Meding B, Swanbeck G: Occupational hand eczema in an industrial city. Contact Dermatitis 22:13–23, 1990.
10. Nethercott JR, Holness DL, Adams RM, et al: Patch testing with a routine screening tray in North America 1985 through 1989. IV. Occupation and response. Am J Contact Dermatitis 2:247–254, 1991.
11. Plotnick H: Analysis of 250 consecutively evaluated cases of workers' disability claims for dermatitis. Arch Dermatol 126:782–786, 1990.

12. Sertoli A, Gola M, Martinelli C, et al: Epidemiology of contact dermatitis. Semin Dermatology 8,2:120–126, 1989.
13. Vestey JP, Gawkrodger DJ, Wong W-K, Buxton PK: An analysis of 501 consecutive contact clinic consultations. Contact Dermatitis 15:119–125, 1986.
14. Wall LM, Gebauer KA: Occupational skin disease in Western Australia. Contact Dermatitis 24:101–109, 1991.
15. Wilkinson DS, Budden MG, Hambly EM: A 10-year review of an industrial dermatitis clinic. Contact Dermatitis 6:11–17, 1980.

DANIEL J. HOGAN, MD

THE PROGNOSIS OF OCCUPATIONAL CONTACT DERMATITIS

The prognosis of contact dermatitis is a crucial issue for the affected worker, the treating physician, the company physician, workers' compensation authorities, and society. The prognosis for recovery from contact dermatitis has not changed significantly over the past half century despite the advent of systemic and topical corticosteroids, PUVA, improvements in working conditions, and our increased knowledge of contact dermatitis.[11] This chapter reviews the prognosis of contact dermatitis, discusses practical reasons for the poor prognosis of contact dermatitis, and comments on the appropriate management of occupational contact dermatitis.

OCCUPATIONAL DERMATITIS

Occupational contact dermatitis and non-occupational contact dermatitis have similar prognoses. Occupational dermatoses, 90% of which are contact dermatitis, account for 30% of occupational disease in the United States. The percentage of reportable occupational illness caused by skin disease has decreased in recent years.[22] The number of workdays lost because of occupational dermatitis has also declined.[2] This appears to reflect improvements in working conditions rather than a change in the natural history of contact dermatitis once clinical dermatitis has occurred. Workers disabled by contact dermatitis do benefit more from intense investigation and rehabilitation than do patients disabled by other chronic skin diseases such as severe congenital ichthyosis or refractory psoriasis.[17] Workers with contact dermatitis are usually younger than workers with other occupational diseases. This facilitates reeducation and retraining of the affected worker but makes early retirement of a worker because of occupational dermatitis impractical.

HAND DERMATITIS

Occupational contact dermatitis most commonly affects the hands, which represent the body site most intensely exposed to occupational skin irritants and allergens and are so crucial to workers, from cleaning staff to surgeons.[2] The majority of workers with occupational hand dermatitis should be patch tested to standard and occupational allergens by a dermatologist with special expertise and training. The need for patch testing is greatest for workers with the most severe dermatitis.[10]

TIME OFF WORK

Some workers with mild hand dermatitis of occupational origin may not require time off work. Other workers may require up to three weeks off work to allow their dermatitis to respond to treatment and to heal. Workers with moderate hand dermatitis often require up to one month of time off work. Workers with severe hand dermatitis usually require two to ten weeks of time off work, and some never fully recover. Practitioners in European countries, particularly Scandinavian countries, recommend a longer period of time off work for occupational hand dermatitis than is customary in North America.[10] The policy may reflect differences in workers' compensation and social welfare laws. It is clear both on clinical experience and on basic immunologic investigations that both irritant and allergic contact dermatitis may precipitate a self-perpetuating cycle of dermatitis.

IRRITANT CONTACT DERMATITIS

People vary in their susceptibility to mild and moderate cutaneous irritants. Those with a past history of atopic hand dermatitis are highly susceptible to cutaneous irritants and suffer most from chronic hand dermatitis.[20]

Cumulative irritant contact dermatitis has the worst prognosis. Acute irritant contact dermatitis affects virtually anyone exposed to a strong cutaneous irritant. This condition has a better prognosis because its occurrence does not require heightened susceptibility of a worker to develop dermatitis. Irritant occupational contact dermatitis to cutting oils is frequent among machinists but usually does not lead to severe disabling dermatitis.[19]

Persistent exposure to irritants at home may cause dermatitis to persist, as it may be easier for some workers to avoid exposure to irritants at work than at home. Other family members may not wish to take over household tasks, and workers who are off work because of dermatitis have more time at home and may increase their exposure to cutaneous irritants at home.

Workers may moonlight at a second job, which may not be covered by workers' compensation and may be unknown to the physician.[23] That second job may be the source of dermatitis rather than the job listed on the insurance or history form.

ALLERGIC CONTACT DERMATITIS

The prognosis for patients with allergic contact dermatitis varies with the contact allergen. Allergic contact dermatitis to nickel or chromate is associated with a poor prognosis for complete healing, particularly in Europe.[23] Allergic contact dermatitis to chemicals added to rubber (e.g., allergic contact dermatitis to rubber gloves used at work), has a good prognosis once the allergy is identified and an appropriate allergen substitution recommended (e.g., work gloves that do not contain the sensitizer to which the worker is allergic). Allergic contact dermatitis to epoxy in high-technology workers usually has a good prognosis.[7] These workers are typically young and their work site is usually cleaner than work sites of the past.

JOB CHANGES

Most workers who have to change jobs because of occupational contact dermatitis suffer significant loss of income.[1] Most workers, even those with severe occupational hand dermatitis, do not have to change occupations. It is clear that a change in occupation is indicated only for a small minority of affected workers.[9,11,15] Workers who may require a job change include those with a severe allergy to a workplace allergen where indirect and direct contact with the allergen cannot be curtailed. Workers with atopic hand dermatitis exacerbated by cutaneous irritants will do better if they can switch to work in which there is no exposure to cutaneous irritants such as water, soaps, and solvents.

Most workers do best if they continue to work for their current employer, recognizing that they may miss brief periods of work for severe flare-ups of their dermatitis. It is preferable for a worker to continue to work at a work site where he or she knows the irritants and allergens that exacerbate the dermatitis and what measures to follow to avoid contact with them.

CHIEF REASONS FOR PERSISTENCE

Misdiagnosis

Most cases of chronic hand dermatitis are due to cutaneous irritants, not allergens. There is no diagnostic test to prove that irritant contact dermatitis in a worker is due to a particular irritant. The diagnosis rests on exclusion of allergic contact dermatitis by careful patch testing for possible workplace and household allergens, the occurrence of dermatitis at a site of direct skin contact with the irritant, and the exclusion of endogenous dermatoses such as psoriasis or a disorder that may masquerade as hand dermatitis such as tinea manus. Irritant contact dermatitis is largely a diagnosis of exclusion, and undiagnosed allergic contact dermatitis may be mislabeled irritant contact dermatitis. Irritant contact dermatitis, allergic contact dermatitis, and endogenous eczema of the hands cannot be distinguished on morphologic grounds.[4]

Continued Exposure to Irritants

Persistent exposure to irritants at work is a major cause of the persistence of hand dermatitis. Workers such as machinists are constantly exposed to irritants such as cutting oils. Housewives, particularly mothers of young children, are exposed to irritants throughout the day and night.[16] Frequent hand washing is required in many occupations such as nursing.

Inappropriate skin cleansing is an important remedial cause of contact dermatitis. Workers must be advised not to wash their hands with abrasive soaps or solvents such as gasoline. No inspection of a work site is complete until the physician examines the washing facilities, as this may reveal inadequate facilities or various abrasive cleaners and solvents used to remove workplace soil from the hands.[13]

Iatrogenic Contact Dermatitis

This is an important remedial cause of occupational hand dermatitis.[14] First-aid departments should not treat workers with potential topical allergens such as neomycin. Many topical corticosteroid preparations contain irritants such as propylene glycol. Workers often do better if treated with corticosteroids in a simple ointment base such as Synalar or Cyclocort ointments. Barrier creams are often irritants themselves and contain potential allergens such as preservatives and fragrances.[11]

Atopy

Atopic hand dermatitis has a poor prognosis. Some individuals with a past history of atopic dermatitis may have a period of remission during late childhood and adolescence only to have their atopic hand dermatitis become unmasked by entering a profession such as hairdressing, in which there is a high risk of occupational irritant contact dermatitis. Individuals with atopic dermatitis should be advised at an early age that they are at increased risk to develop irritant contact dermatitis if they enter occupations such as hairdressing or nursing, in which exposure to cutaneous irritants is chronic and unavoidable.

Chronicity

The risk of chronic dermatitis increases with the severity of the hand dermatitis. The pathogenesis of chronic, self-perpetuating dermatitis is unresolved.[12] It is hoped that further research into the pathogenesis of dermatitis, particularly the immunology of irritant as well as allergic contact dermatitis, will lead to the development of treatment modalities that can arrest this destructive, self-perpetuating cycle. It is clear that the strongest predictive factor for future dermatitis is a history of chronic dermatitis.[8] Occupational health physicians are well aware that the longer a worker is off work, the less likely a worker is to return to work.

Continued Exposure to Allergens

Persistent allergen exposure at work is another important cause of chronic occupational contact dermatitis. Infrequent intermittent exposure to an allergen at work (e.g., once every 2–3 weeks) can account for persistent dermatitis. An occupational history from workers must critically review not only workers' daily exposure to irritants and allergens but also their exposure to materials used episodically such as during retooling, major overhauls, and cleaning times at work. Only careful investigation of a patient's dermatitis can identify the allergens at work. Many allergens remain to be identified and will not be detected by patch testing to the limited number of allergens on the U.S. Food and Drug Administration–approved standard tray available through the American Academy of Dermatology.

Insufficient Advice to Patients

We are limited by our lack of knowledge of all the possible sources of exposure to occupational allergens. It is clear that the more the patient knows about relevant irritants and allergens, the better the prognosis.[5] Workers vary in their intelligence and in their compliance with allergen avoidance.

Nondermatologic Factors

When one evaluates a patient with hand dermatitis, one is evaluating more than the patient's epidermis. Factors such as depression, problems with coworkers, pressing family responsibilities, and low pay may all impede a worker's ability to return to work.[17,21]

Endogenous Hand Dermatitis

Even experienced dermatologists cannot accurately distinguish clinically endogenous hand dermatitis from either irritant or allergic occupational hand dermatitis. Because its onset is unrelated to an irritant or allergen at work, the course of endogenous hand dermatitis is unaffected by modifications of workplace exposures. There is a tendency for workers to ascribe to the workplace the origin of their dermatitis of endogenous origin.[18] Once their dermatitis has been labeled occupational in origin, it is difficult to dissuade workers from this conviction.

Multifactorial Hand Dermatitis

Hand dermatitis does not represent a specific diagnosis, but it is nevertheless a useful term regarding therapy and advice to the patient.[6] Hand dermatitis is frequently multifactorial in origin.[3] For example, a worker with irritant contact dermatitis of the hands from frequent hand washing or exposure to solvents may start to wear rubber gloves to protect the hands. Eventually, that worker may become sensitized to one of the preservatives found in the rubber gloves and then develop allergic contact dermatitis to the rubber gloves. Diagnosis of this allergy and subsequent allergen avoidance will reduce the severity of the hand dermatitis and make it easier to treat, but the dermatitis may not resolve entirely until the underlying irritant contact dermatitis is managed optimally.

PATCH TESTING

Patch testing plays a crucial role in the evaluation of patients with occupational hand dermatitis. The worker must be patch tested for all relevant allergens to which he or she is exposed at work and at home. One must remember that a positive patch test reaction proves only that a patient is allergic to a chemical. A positive reaction does not prove that a patient's dermatitis is caused by that chemical. Both the patient's history and the practitioner's clinical knowledge are also required to accurately diagnose allergic contact dermatitis.

It is hoped that further research into the pathogenesis and treatment of contact dermatitis will lead to a real change in the prognosis of workers with contact dermatitis of the hands.

REFERENCES

1. Burrows D: Prognosis in industrial dermatitis. Br J Dermatol 87:145–148, 1972.
2. Church R: Hand eczema in industry and the home. In Griffiths WAD, Wilkinson DS (eds): Essentials of Industrial Dermatology. Oxford, Blackwell, 1985, pp 85–100.
3. Coenraads PJ: Prevalence of hand eczema: Association with occupational exposure, especially in construction workers. Groningen, Krips Repro Meppel, 1983.
4. Cronin E: Clinical patterns of hand eczema in women. Contact Dermatitis 13:153–161, 1985.
5. Edman B: The usefulness of detailed information to patients with contact allergy. Contact Dermatitis 19:43–47, 1988.
6. Epstein E: Hand dermatitis: Practical management and current concepts. J Am Acad Dermatol 10:395–424, 1984.
7. Fregert S: Occupational dermatitis in a 10-year material. Contact Dermatitis 1:96–107, 1975.

8. Gallant CJ: A long term follow-up study of patients with hand dermatitis evaluated at St. Michael's Occupational Health Clinic in 1981 and 1982. Master's Thesis, 1986.
9. Hellier FF: The prognosis in industrial dermatitis. Br Med J 1:196–198, 1958.
10. Hogan DJ, Dannaker CJ, Lal S, Maibach HI: An international survey of expert opinion on the prognosis of contact dermatitis. Dermatosen in Beruf und Umwelt 38:143–147, 1990.
11. Hogan DJ, Dannaker CJ, Maibach HI: The prognosis of contact dermatitis. J Am Acad Dermatol 23:300–307, 1990.
12. Markey AC, Allen MH, Pitzalis C, MacDonald DM: T-cell inducer populations in cutaneous inflammation: A predominance of T-helper-inducer lymphocytes (THI) in the infiltrate of inflammatory dermatoses. Br J Dermatol 122:325–332, 1990.
13. Mathias CGT: Contact dermatitis from use or misuse of soaps, detergents, and cleansers in the workplace. Occup Med State Art Rev 1:205–218, 1986.
14. Morris GE: Why doesn't the worker's skin clear up? Arch Indust Hyg 10:43–44, 1954.
15. Nethercott JR: Disability due to occupational contact dermatitis. Occup Med 1:199–203, 1986.
16. Nilsson E, Mikaelsson B, Anderson S: Atopy, occupation and domestic work as risk factors for hand eczema in hospital workers. Contact Dermatitis 13:216–223, 1985.
17. O'Quinn SE, Cole J, Many H: Problems of disability and rehabilitation in patients with chronic skin diseases. Arch Dermatol 105:35–41, 1972.
18. Phillips B: Occupational dermatitis. Practitioner 172:531–537, 1954.
19. Pryce DW, Irvine D, English JSC, Rycroft RJG: Soluble oil dermatitis: A follow-up study. Contact Dermatitis 21:28–35, 1989.
20. Rystedt I: Hand eczema and long term prognosis in atopic dermatitis. Acta Dermatol Venereol 117:1–59, 1985.
21. Taylor P: Aspects of sickness absence. In Gardner AW (ed): Current Approaches to Occupational Medicine. Bristol, John Wright & Sons, 1979, pp 322–338.
22. U.S. Bureau of Labor Statistics: Occupational injuries and illnesses in the United States by industry–1983. Department of Labor Bulletin 2236:56, 1985.
23. Wilkinson DS: Causes of unexpected persistence of an occupational dermatitis. In Griffiths WAD, Wilkinson DS (eds): Essentials of Industrial Dermatology. Oxford, Blackwell, 1985, pp 111–124.

CHESTER L. DAVIDSON, MD

OCCUPATIONAL CONTACT DERMATITIS OF THE UPPER EXTREMITY

The physician caring for patients in an industrial environment is apt to see a wide variety of occupational diseases. However, more workers suffer from occupational skin diseases than from any other single category of work-related disorder.[39] Mathias[23] reported that approximately 40% of all work-related conditions involve the skin. Between 90 and 95% of occupational skin diseases are contact dermatitis in origin, and more than one-third of them involve the hand and upper extremity.

About 25% of workers with occupational skin disease lose time from work. Each worker affected misses an average of 10–12 workdays because of such a disease.[23] The consequences of occupational contact dermatitis to the worker can be even more serious than loss of time from work. Contact dermatitis may force the employee to lose a seniority position or even to change careers.

Once the physician determines that the workers' dermatitis is of contact origin, whether or not the causation is occupational must be established by determining whether the worker was exposed to the offending agent in the workplace. Both the employee and the employer benefit from these determinations. If the causation is occupational, frequently the problem can be eliminated. The employee can reduce the number of workdays missed, and the employer can decrease the amount of production lost due to occupational illness. Once an occupational basis of the worker's dermatitis is established, the employer must address the additional issue

OCCUPATIONAL MEDICINE: State of the Art Reviews—
Vol. 9, No. 1, January–March 1994. Philadelphia, Hanley & Belfus, Inc.

of safety in the workplace and may be required to assume additional financial responsibilities.

A comprehensive review of occupational skin diseases is beyond the scope of this chapter and can be found in texts[2,9,13] and periodicals dedicated to this subject (e.g., *Contact Dermatitis* and the *American Journal of Contact Dermatitis.*) General emphasis here will be placed on irritant, allergic, and urticarial contact dermatitis. Recent findings will be related to specific occupations whose workers are at increased risk of developing contact dermatitis of the hand and upper extremity. Harmful materials to which the worker is exposed will be enumerated, and methods useful for peventing or reducing contact with noxious substances in the workplace will be detailed. A section on workers' compensation will delineate criteria useful in determining whether the worker's contact dermatitis is of occupational origin.

TYPES OF DERMATITIS

Contact with chemicals constitutes the major dermatological hazard in the working population. Each year the introduction of new compounds and processes broadens the hazardous potential.[6] Contact with many chemical substances, both organic and inorganic, causes various types of dermatitis. Most of these substances produce irritant contact dermatitis; some cause allergic contact dermatitis; and contact with a few causes contact urticaria.

Contact dermatitis is a reactive inflammation in the skin provoked by direct contact with environmental chemicals or substances.[24] The morphology of irritant and allergic contact dermatitis is mostly nonspecific, but eczematous changes are typically found. There are no morphological or histological features that reliably allow the clinician to distinguish between irritant and allergic origins of the worker's dermatitis. Patch testing may be required to differentiate these types of contact dermatitis.

Hand dermatitis can be seriously disabling and is often chronic. Its management can be frustrating even to the most experienced physician. Regardless of the etiology of hand dermatitis (allergic or irritant contact dermatitis, atopic eczema, psoriasis, or other), nonspecific irritation, both in the work environment and at home, is frequently a factor in aggravating and continuing the dermatitis. For example, once the skin's barrier function has been compromised by overuse or improper use of skin cleaning agents, exposure to solvents, or other cause, the skin is susceptible to the effects of these and many other environmental materials.

Irritant contact dermatitis (Figs. 1–3) is produced by materials that act directly on the skin via nonimmunological mechanisms.[2] The application of chemical substances produces irritant dermatitis initially by disrupting the skin's barrier. Irritation develops predominantly or exclusively on skin surfaces that come into obvious, frequent, or repeated contact with the causal agent. The distribution of the dermatitis depends somewhat on the physical form of the causal agent and the manner in which exposure occurs. Contact with solids and liquids causes an eruption on the exposed areas, commonly the hands and the upper extremity; contact with fumes, vapors, or mists, on the other hand, causes an eruption on all exposed areas such as the face, ears, neck, and upper extremity.[11] Because the palmar surfaces are relatively resistant to irritant dermatitis, the site of initial hand involvement may be the finger webs or the dorsal surfaces of the hands. The dermatitis may progress to involve the entire hand and upper extremity.

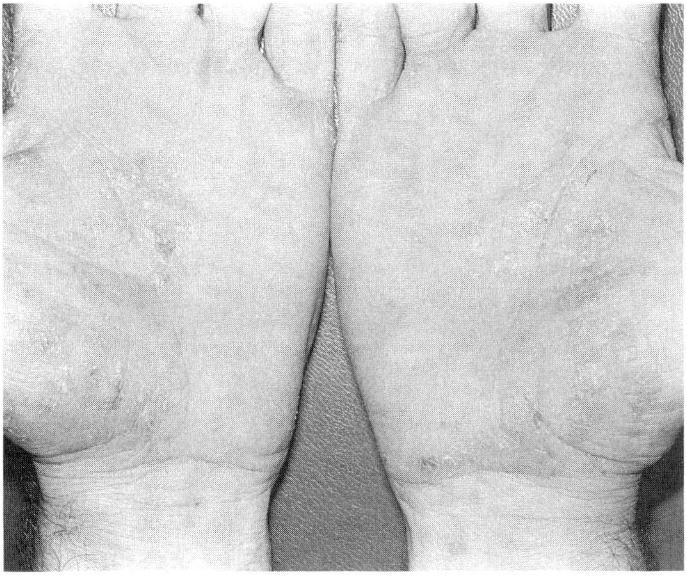

FIGURE 1. An irritant dermatitis on the hands of a furniture finisher resulting from cleanup with solvents.

A diagnosis of irritant dermatitis is based on a clinical history of exposure to a known potential irritant and on physical findings of appropriate skin changes in expected locations. The clinical appearance of dermatitis varies considerably depending on the type and duration of the exposure. Only slight erythema may result from contact with a mild irritant. Moderately irritating substances produce an eczematous reaction characterized by erythema, vesiculation with subsequent

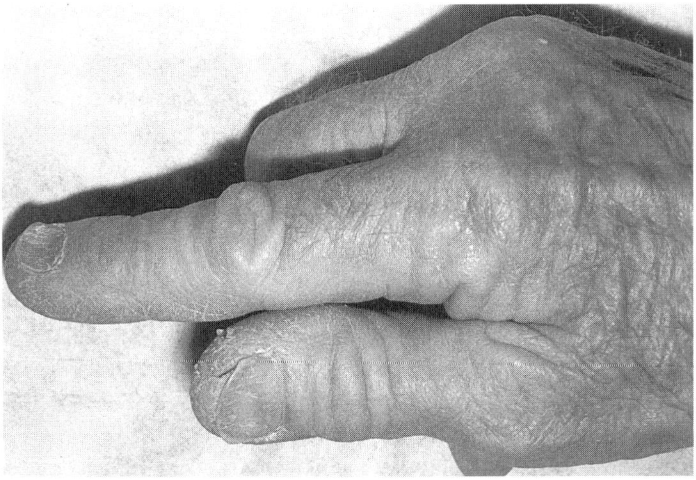

FIGURE 2. Xerotic irritant dermatitis and occupational koilonychia (spoon nail) in a painter who used mineral spirits for cleanup.

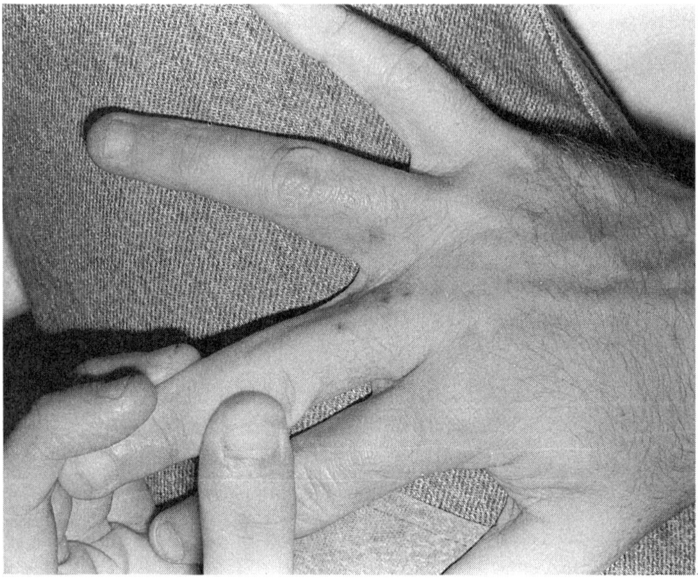

FIGURE 3. The hands of a slaugherhouse worker who developed macerated irritant dermatitis from wet work while processing picnic hams.

oozing, crusting, and scaling.[2] Large bullae with necrosis and ulceration may result from contact with a strong irritant.

Weaker irritants, such as detergents or solvents may produce dermatitis only after repeated or prolonged exposures. A strong irritant such as battery acid, however, rapidly causes a demonstrable reaction in the majority of people on first exposure. The patient with irritant dermatitis may report stinging and burning sensations. Pruritus is variable and not usually as severe as in the vesicular stages of allergic contact dermatitis.[2]

Given the necessary environmental conditions and exposures, any chemical or substance may be a potential irritant. Many factors cause a substance to become an irritant, including inherent chemical properties, application site, and duration of exposure. Friction, occlusion, local trauma, heat, humidity, and ultraviolet light are important factors contributing to the production of irritant contact dermatitis. Some common agents capable of causing irritant contact dermatitis in the workplace are shown in Table 1

The most important risk factors predisposing the worker to irritant dermatitis are considered to be atopy and other preexisting skin disease.[23] Several studies demonstrate that atopic persons are at higher risk for developing irritant contact dermatitis.[21,31] Individuals with existing allergic or irritant dermatitis also have a lowered threshold for further irritation probably because of disruption of the skin's

TABLE 1. Common Industrial Irritants[23]

Detergents	Food substances
Solvents	Plants
Petroleum oils and grease	Fiberglass and other particulate dust
Machining (cutting) fluids and lubricants	

barrier.[7] The importance of the worker's preexisting or underlying dermatitis is discussed in the section on workers' compensation.

Allergic contact dermatitis (ACD) is an acquired immunologically mediated (delayed) inflammatory response in the skin to contact with environmental allergenic substances (Fig. 4). Of the thousands of chemicals in commercial use today, only about 200 are commonly recognized as allergic contact sensitizers.[2] Table 2 lists the most common allergens to which workers are exposed. Only a small percentage of people develop sensitivity to the many allergenic substances in the environment. In addition to personal susceptibility to allergy, the antigen itself may determine the sensitization rate. *Rhus* oleoresin (the exudate causing poison ivy and oak), for example, is able to sensitize about 70% of people exposed.[2]

In contrast to the rapidly evolving eruption resulting from contact with a potent irritating substance, skin lesions in a sensitized individual may not appear for several days to a week after exposure to the offending allergen.[6] Typically ACD begins with erythema, which is followed by papules and vesicles that often rupture and ooze. Interdigital and palmar surfaces initially show multiple pruritic vesicles in groups and clusters.

As with irritant dermatitis, the skin surfaces affected depend on the physical form of the allergen and the manner in which exposure occurs. The distribution of the skin eruption corresponds with that of the antigenic exposure. Involvement of additional skin surfaces without obvious contact, however, is much more likely to occur with contact allergy than with irritant dermatitis.[23] New lesions may appear at distant, unrelated sites owing to inadvertent transfer of the allergen by the hands or through autosensitization "id" type phenomena.[2]

A positive patch test confirms the clinical diagnosis of ACD. Once the presence of the offending allergen is demonstrated in the workplace, employee protection and antigen replacement efforts can begin. Adams and Fisher[4] outline

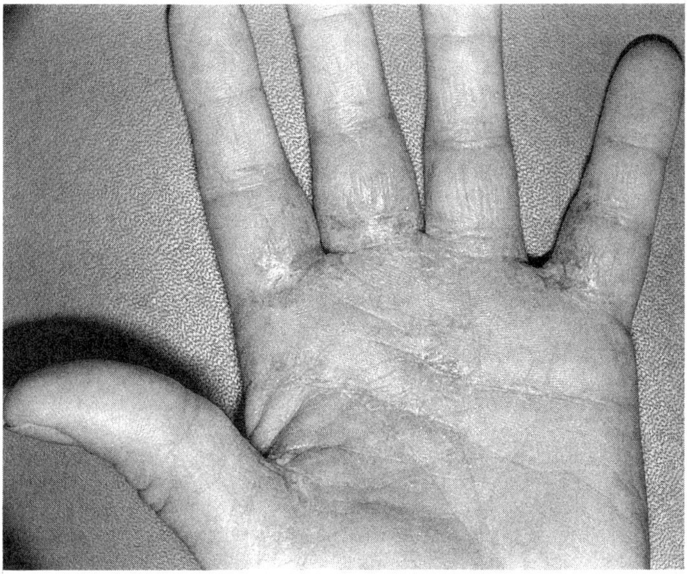

FIGURE 4. Allergic contact dermatitis from lacquer on a cabinetmaker's hands.

TABLE 2. Common Industrial Allergens[11,13,23,35,39]

Rhus and *Compositae* plant species
Metallic salts and compounds of nickel, chromate, cobalt, and gold
Various accelerators and antioxidants used in rubber
Uncured epoxy, acrylic, and phenoformaldehyde resins (including hardeners and curing agents)
Organic dyes (PPDA and like compounds)
Biocides and germicides

safe and practical alternatives for common and important antigens currently encountered industrially. The interested reader will find their comprehensive and detailed treatise invaluable in helping remove the worker from industrial exposure to antigenic substances.

Contact urticaria is a local skin response that occurs at the sites of primary contact with various materials.[23] The reaction generally begins less than 1 hour after exposure. The mode of action of chemical urticariogens is unknown. Both immunological and nonimmunological factors have been implicated.[20,41]

Contact urticaria is usually characterized as a wheal-and-flare response at the site of contact. Taylor,[38] however, found that this response occurs only in some cases and that erythema predominates. Most patients have various transient sensations such as itching, burning, and stinging. Kligman[20] reported that these suburticariogenic responses are often related to the concentration of the offending urticariogen. He found that patients who develop contact urticaria from a specific concentration of an offending substance generally develop only erythema from contact with a diluted amount of the substance and that further dilution variably produces pruritus alone.

Some patients may develop a more generalized reaction with distant or widespread urticarial lesions, perhaps owing to percutaneous absorption. Only rarely is the reaction severe enough to lead to anaphylactic shock.[23,38] In addition to the contact urticarial reaction, many patients also experience irritant or allergic contact dermatitis.

It is likely that contact urticaria occurs more commonly than reports suggest. The transient nature of the eruption makes observation difficult. Likewise, patients who experience only pruritus or erythema at the site of contact with urticariogenic substances may not seek diagnostic evaluation. Nethercott and Holmes[29] established only one case of contact urticaria (in a cook who was sensitive to shellfish) among the 1,346 patients assessed and patch-tested between 1981 and 1988.

Hazardous Occupations

Because the National Institute for Occupational Safety and Health lists dermatological disorders as one of the most common occupational-related conditions, Mathias and Morrison[25] sought to identify current high-risk industries for the development of occupational skin disease. They reviewed the overall rates, numbers, and proportions of occupational skin disease recorded in the Bureau of Labor Statistics Annual Survey of Occupational Injuries and illnesses from 1973 to 1984. Industries with the highest incidences of contact dermatitis are listed in Table 3. Manufacturing (especially of rubber and plastic products) and agricultural industries consistently reported the highest incidences and largest total numbers of

TABLE 3. Industries and Products Associated with High Incidences of Contact Dermatitis[23]

Landscaping and horticulture	Adhesives and sealants
Forestry	Leather tanning and finishing
Poultry dressing and processing	Abrasive products
Fresh and frozen packaged fish	Plating and polishing operations
Beet sugar	Storage batteries
Miscellaneous agricultural chemicals	Boat building and repairing
Surface active agents and penetrants (emulsifiers, wetting agents, finishing oils, etc.)	Ophthalmic goods
	Miscellaneous sporting and athletic goods

workers with contact dermatitis. In fact, skin disease accounted for nearly two-thirds of all occupational illness within the various agricultural industries.

Hazardous Exposures

Storrs et al.[37] compiled the results of patch testing carried out by the North American Contact Dermatitis Group for the years 1984 and 1985. The most common sensitizers identified were nickel, paraphylenediamine (PPDA), quaternium-15, neomycin, thimerosal, formaldehyde, cinnamic aldehyde, and thiuram compounds. Because these substances are found both in the home and the workplace, the results are applicable to patients with both occupation- and non-occupation-related allergic contact dermatitis. In one-third of patients (398 of 1,199) who reacted, the hand was the primary site of dermatitis. Table 4 lists industrial agents that most frequently cause irritant or allergic contact dermatitis.

EXAMPLES

Contact Urticaria

Because contact urticaria is most frequently caused by foods (e.g., dairy products, fish, citrus, fruits, nuts, spices, grains, meats, and vegetables) containing allergens and vasoactive substances, food handlers are at particular risk of developing it.[23] Other occupations at risk include veterinarians and slaughterhouse workers (animal hair and tissue), gardeners (plants and grasses), hairdressers (henna dye[30] and ammonium persulfate[16,19]), and health care workers (medicinals, rubefacients, and allergenic antibiotics[23]). Taylor[38] cited examples including a physician and several patients, one a newborn, who developed contact symptoms of urticaria after exposure to latex gloves. Symptoms of contact urticaria from latex glove exposure range from local itching and redness to alarming and potentially serious systemic reactions such as generalized urticaria, rhinitis, asthma, and even anaphylaxis.[15]

TABLE 4. Substances and Conditions Frequently Causing Occupation-related Contact Dermatitis[1,12]

Poison ivy and oak	Metals and metalic salts
Detergents and cleaning agents	Fiberglass and particulate dust
Solvents	Plastics and resins
Machining oils and coolants	Textiles, fabrics, and related materials
Petroleum oil, greases, and lubricants	Infectious agents
Food products	Rubbish, dirt, and sewage
Inedible plants or animals	Environmental conditions (heat and humidity)
Agricultural chemicals	

Irritant and Allergic Contact Dermatitis

Because they handle many irritating and allergenic substances, workers in certain occupations are at particular risk of developing contact dermatitis of the hand and upper extremity. Food handlers, hairdressers, and various horticulturists will be discussed here with particular reference to recently published findings.

Food Handlers

Fisher[13] categorizes dermatitis resulting from contact with foods into five varieties: (1) irritant dermatitis, (2) allergic contact dermatitis, (3) immediate urticarial type of dermatitis (contact urticaria), (4) immediate vesicular eruption, and (5) phototoxic dermatitis. Foods such as citruses are capable of producing all these reactions. Other foods are notorious for causing a particular reaction; contact with celery and limes, for example, causes phytophototoxic dermatitis.

Certain plants contain light-sensitizing compounds that cause irritant dermatitis upon skin exposure to certain wavelengths of ultraviolet light (phytophototoxic dermatitis).[5] Furanocoumarin compounds, for example, are found in the *Umbelliferae* family (celery, parsley, carrots, and coriander), the *Moraceae* family (common figs), and the *Rutaceae* family (limes, common rue, burning bush, hog-wood plant, among others). These phytoalexins are produced by the plant in response to disease or injury, and they probably contribute to the plant's disease resistance. Exposure to these plant families commonly causes blistering erythematous lesions with or without postinflammatory hyperpigmentation.

Celery is one of the major causes of phytophotodermatitis in farmers who harvest it and in industrial workers who process the plant stalks and leaves. Berkley et al.[5] described 30 grocery store workers who developed a phytophototoxic dermatitis from celery. The eruption was vesicular and scaly and occurred mostly on the dorsum of the hands, interdigital areas, and inner aspect of the forearms. It was often linear as a result of brushing contact with the plant, which streaked the furanocoumarin across the skin.

Bartenders commonly develop vesicular phytophotodermatitis on the first and second fingers from squeezing limes while making cocktails outdoors in the summer months. Workers engaged in collecting figs and bergamot fruit commonly develop hyperpigmentation of the hands without antecedent dermatitis.[5]

Exposure to citrus fruit is increased in certain occupations, including the citrus growing and packaging industries, food and beverage preparation (such as cooks, bakers, and bartenders), and retail food sales. Citrus handlers develop allergic contact reactions to peel oil (D-limonene, geraniol, and citral) and irritant dermatitis from contact with fruit juices.[8] Other contact dermatitis reactions are seen in workers exposed to extraneous allergens and irritants applied to the fruit. These substances include dyes, wax coatings, fertilizers, and mold-retarding agents.[8] The hands are most often the site of citrus allergic or irritant dermatitis.[9]

Hand dermatitis from chromates is a frequent problem among cement workers, foundry workers and welders, sheet metal workers, those who work in offset printing, and, recently, workers in the milk-producing industry.[17] Potassium dichromate is used to preserve a milk sample for transportation from the farm to the quality control laboratory for assay for protein, butterfat, and white blood cells (an indicator of bovine mastitis). In a Pennsylvania quality control laboratory that examines 300,000 samples of milk monthly, Herzog et al.[17] found that the use of chromates as preservatives places laboratory workers exposed at considerable risk for developing allergic contact dermatitis. Antigen substitutions with bronopol and Kathon CG (methylisothiazolinone) are recommended in order to reduce the incidence of allergic contact dermatitis among workers in milk-testing laboratories.

HAIRDRESSERS

The principal occupational cutaneous hazard for hairdressers is contact dermatitis. Hairdressers repeatedly come into contact with a variety of substances, including hair tonics, permanent wave solutions, dyes, and shampoos. Exposure to these chemicals while doing their usually wet work makes the occurrence of irritant, allergic, and urticarial contact dermatitis a well-recognized occupational disease among hairdressers.[30] Hairdressers' contact dermatitis is most often of an irritant nature.[18] In some cases, hand dermatitis improves merely by virtue of the beautician's being promoted out of frequent hair washing.

The most common sensitizers that hairdressers are exposed to are PPDA (hair dyes), nickel (metal accessories), thiuram compounds (rubber gloves), formaldehyde (shampoos), thioglycolates (permanent wave solutions), and ammonium persulfate (bleaches).[13,14,16,18,19]

Nethercott et al.[30] patch-tested 18 hairdressers who had hand dermatitis and confirmed that PPDA compounds in hair dyes are by far the most common sensitizers. Typically, the ACD that results from contact with these dyes begins on the medial aspect of the index and middle fingers used to hold the hair to be dyed.

Many hairdressers have been forced to change occupations because of PPDA allergy. In one series only 37.5% of the hairdressers with PPDA allergies were able to continue work in the trade.[30] It is possible, however, that advising a hairdresser who is sensitive to PPDA to seek other employment is ill advised. Reiss and Fisher[33] found that hair properly dyed with PPDA is not allergenic. PPDA-sensitized hairdressers can handle PPDA-dyed hair and can usually apply PPDA dye to their clients' hair without being subject to hand dermatitis if they wear gloves. Vinyl gloves are preferred because of the hairdressers increased risk of becoming sensitized to rubber gloves.[13] Hairdressers and others who are known to be allergic to PPDA should be informed about possible allergic cross-reactions with benzocaine, procaine, sulfonamides, and sunscreens containing para-aminobenzoic acid (PABA).[13]

Glyceryl monothioglycolate (GMTG), a common sensitizer of both hairdressers and their clients,[42] is a reducing agent used in "acid" or "hot" salon permanent waves.[36] Ammonium thioglycolate is used under alkaline conditions for "cold" permanent waves. It is considered an irritant and, rarely, a sensitizer.[13,18] Morrison and Storrs[27] demonstrated the persistence of GMTG antigen in hair at least 3 months after the use of permanent wave solutions. The persistence of this compound may explain the long-lasting dermatitis that occurs in hairdressers and clients sensitive to GMTG.

The use of heavy rubber gloves while administering a "hot" salon permanent has been shown to protect sensitized hairdressers from reacting while applying GMTG to the hair. These gloves, however, are often too cumbersome to be of practical use.[36] Until a lightweight effective barrier glove is introduced, it would be best for sensitized hairdressers to avoid applying permanent wave solutions or to use "cold" hair permanents, if they are not also allergic to ammonium thioglycolate. Because of the persistence of GMTG antigens in the hair, GMTG-sensitive hairdressers should wear protective gloves when shampooing or otherwise handling hair that has been treated with GMTG.

Ammonium persulfate is used in hair bleaches as an oxidizer to boost peroxide bleaches and accelerate the bleaching process.[18] It is known to cause irritant dermatitis, ACD, and contact urticaria in hairdressers. Because Kellett and Beck[19] found positive patch tests to ammonium persulfate in 25% of hairdressers (12 of 49) who presented with hand dermatitis, it appears that ammonium persulfate is also a relatively common sensitizer of hairdressers.

Hairdressers' occupational health and safety can be improved by making them aware of their potential for allergy and by changes in their work habits. They should be encouraged to eliminate as many allergens as possible from the workplace and to use gloves when working with various chemicals. Hairdressers need to wash and rinse their hands more often and to use emollients frequently.

Horticulturists

In the United States contact dermatitis due to wild vegetation is caused most commonly by plants of the *Compositae* (daisy) and *Rhus* (poison ivy) families.[26] Although poison ivy remains the most frequent and important cause of phytodermatitis, the investigator should be aware of the important role other plants play in producing contact dermatitis.

Menz and Winkelman[26] patch-tested 74 patients suspected of having dermatitis to wild vegetation other than to *Rhus.* The eruption produced was typically similar to the acute ACD resulting from *Rhus* exposure. About three-quarters of cases were localized, and more than 90% affected an extremity. Dog fennel and cocklebur gave the most frequent positive patch-test results. Less frequent reactions were found with cedar, juniper, wild feverfew, fleabane, and burweed marsh elder. Gardening was the most common source of exposure to weeds.

Hand dermatitis represents a significant problem in the floral industry; about 45,000 workers are at risk in the United States.[40] Contact dermatitis in floral workers results from exposure to soaps, detergents, water, fertilizers, herbicides, and irritating or allergenic plants.[1] *Alstroemeria* (Peruvian or Inca lily) and *Chrysanthemum* are probably the most common plants causing ACD among flower shop workers.[40] *Alstroemeria* was introduced into floral design in the United States in about 1981 and is a particular favorite of florists because of its longlasting beauty. The hand dermatitis produced is often chronic and associated with scaling and fissuring of the tips of the fingers, which come into prolonged or repeated contact with the stems and petals. The eruption is similar to the ACD *(tulip fingers)* that involves the forefinger and thumbs of tulip bulb workers. *Alstroemeria* and tulips share a common antigen (tuliposide A).[3,40]

Wearing gloves when exposed to *Alstroemeria* may offer protection, but Marks[22] noted that tuliposide A penetrates vinyl, but not nitrile latex, gloves. However, the presence of the juice of the plant on scissors, clippers, table tops, vases, and other work surfaces makes contact with tuliposide A almost impossible to avoid. In many cases, the dermatitis is so severe that the worker has to change jobs.[3]

PREVENTING CONTACT DERMATITIS

General Measures

The effects of extrinsic environmental factors on the skin are mostly preventable through recognition, education, and avoidance of provocative agents.[43] Contact dermatitis is mostly prevented by protection from, or removal of, potential irritants and allergens from the work environment. The employee's work surfaces should be kept clean to avoid contamination of these areas. Irritants, allergens, or other noxious agents should be removed from the skin as soon as possible after contact occurs.

Educating the worker in the proper use of potential irritants found in the workplace will help the employee avoid dermatitis. For example, abrasive cleaners strip off superficial layers of the skin. Because continued use may adversely affect the skin's barrier function, abrasive cleaners should be restricted to thick palmar skin.[23] Waterless cleaners contain solvents that dissolve oily substances that soil the skin. Overuse leads to defatting the skin, which makes the skin more susceptible to dermatitis. The use of waterless cleansers should be followed by gently washing with a mild hand soap and water to remove any residual film. Repeated applications of a skin moisturizer may be helpful to retard any irritating effects of repeated washings with relatively harsh workplace cleaners.

Certain environmental conditions should be avoided in the workplace because exposure to them adds to the disruption of the skin's barrier function and increases the incidence of irritant dermatitis. Included are low relative humidity, friction, pressure, traction, and localized trauma, such as abrasion.[34,43] Combining the drying effects of low ambient air, low water temperature, and low relative humidity may result in chapping and dermatitis. Overhydration of the skin during wet work not only creates problems of maceration and irritation but also predisposes the skin to infections with bacteria, yeasts, and fungi.[43]

Protective Clothing

Efforts should be directed to ways, such as the use of protective clothing and devices, of preventing exposure of the worker to industrial substances.[43] Protective clothing must be properly designed for the task to be performed and fitted to the individual. Clothing and devices used for worker protection may themselves cause ACD. Included are gloves, fingerstalls, boots, safety shoes, masks, safety spectacles, helmets, and aprons.[15] Because the clothing may aggravate as well as cause a dermatitis, care must be taken to reduce heat entrapment and frictional irritation of the skin. Clothing may trap moisture and occlude potentially damaging substances next to the skin for prolonged periods and increase the likelihood that dermatitis will develop (Fig. 5)

Workers can usually protect their hands from direct contact with various industrial chemicals by wearing waterproof, heavy-duty vinyl gloves. In order to adequately protect the worker, gloves must have appropriate chemical and physical resistance and sufficient flexibility for the job task to be performed.[23] Gloves can provide effective protection from contact with irritants and from most allergens, but care must be taken to ensure that allergens do not pass through various glove materials in sufficient amounts to provoke an allegic contact dermatitis.[28,40] Vinyl gloves are often recommended for worker protection because of the smaller incidence of sensitization to vinyl.[13] The use of rubber gloves to protect workers who currently have dermatitis is potentially a therapeutic nightmare. Because the skin's barrier is disrupted, the worker's dermatitis can be complicated by the development of a secondary allergic contact dermatitis from various allergenic rubber compounds in the gloves.

Barrier Creams

The effectiveness of barrier creams for skin protection is controversial and unsupported by clinical trials.[1,23,32] To provide the worker with good protection,

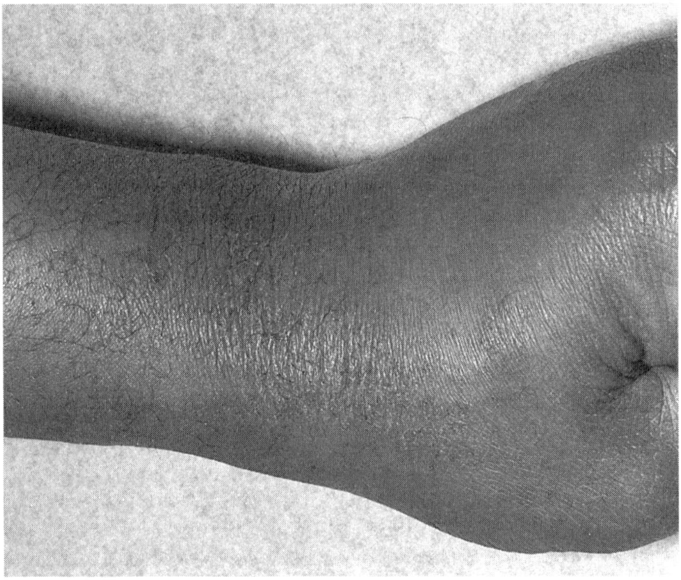

FIGURE 5. The wrist of a slaughterhouse worker who developed an irritant contact dermatitis from hog blood and body fluids trapped under the cuff of his rubber glove.

the barrier cream should increase the skin's barrier function and make it impossible for allergens or irritating substances to penetrate the skin. At most, the cream's effects last only minutes, and the worker needs to reapply the cream frequently to ensure continued protection. If no other means of protection is available, a barrier cream may be used, but its composition must match the job to be done. A water-repellent type should be chosen for defense against acids, alkalies, water-soluble substances, soaps, and detergents. An oil-repellent cream is needed to protect against oils and organic solvents.[2] Because the skin usually tolerates barrier creams well, the creams are often very useful to facilitate the removal of oils and greases from the skin.[23] However, cost considerations usually prevent routine use except in workers with sensitive skin.

WORKERS' COMPENSATION

Contact dermatitis accounts for more than 90% of all workers' compensation claims from occupational skin diseases. About 80% of these claims are attributed to cutaneous irritation. Contact allergy accounts for most of the remainder.[13]

Workers' compensation laws in all states require only reasonable probability (more than 50% likelihood) that the employee's dermatitis resulted directly from occupational exposure. Mathias[24] modified general criteria used to determine probable occupational causation of any skin disease and applied them to contact dermatitis (Table 5). Reasonable probability can be determined by the examining physician after finding positive correlation of the worker's medical history and cutaneous findings with at least four of the seven criteria presented in Table 5.

TABLE 5. Criteria for Evaluating Probable Occupational Causation in Contact Dermatitis[24]

1. The clinical appearance of the worker's dermatitis is consistent with that of a contact dermatitis.
2. The worker is exposed at the workplace to potential cutaneous irritants or allergens.
3. The anatomic distribution of the worker's dermatitis is consistent with cutaneous exposure in relation to the job task.
4. The temporal relationship between exposure and onset is consistent with contact dermatitis.
5. Nonoccupational exposures are excluded as probable causes.
6. The dermatitis improves when the worker is not exposed to the suspected irritant or allergen.
7. Patch tests identify a probable causal agent.

Discussion of Criteria

Criterion 1. Contact dermatitis is clinically an inflammatory eczematous process. As the worker's dermatitis progresses from acute to chronic stages, the clinical findings change from acute vesiculation to subacute serous exudation, from scaling and early lichenification to chronic scaling and predominant lichenification.

Although the skin biopsy demonstrates an eczematous inflammatory response, it is important to realize that the histological findings do not demonstrate the actual cause of the eczematization or whether it is related to an occupation.

Criterion 2. In obtaining a history of the evolution of the dermatitic process, important data must be documented concerning the employee's current job and how he does it. The history should also include:

1. Determination of the employee's exposure to industrial substances
2. Cleanup procedures, including materials used (soaps, solvents, soapless cleaners, abrasives, and so forth)
3. Previous treatment used by the worker (By determining preparations used to treat the dermatitis the examiner may be able to identify a secondary allergic contact dermatitis.)
4. Availability and use of protective clothing such as gloves, sleeves, and aprons.

Criterion 3. Skin surfaces that are maximally exposed develop the most contact dermatitis. For example, dermatitis from industrial liquids occurs on the hands and upper extremities, where direct contact is most frequent. If the distribution of the employee's dermatitis does not match the industrial exposure, a relationship cannot be formed. An example of a negative relationship would be the development of psoriasis in areas free from industrial mechanical trauma or the development of tinea pedis in a factory worker whose feet remain dry on the job.

Criterion 4. With the exception of skin exposures to strong irritants, a lag period is usually seen from beginning an exposure to a substance to erupting with either an allergic or irritant contact dermatitis. Sufficient time is needed for the irritant to interrupt the skin's barrier or the antigen to induce an allergic reaction. The lag period extends from a few weeks to several months and generally does not exceed 6 months.

Criterion 5. Nonoccupational causes of the employee's dermatitis must be excluded by means of the worker's history and by patch testing when indicated or appropriate.

Criterion 6. A weekend away from work or even a few days off from work are usually insufficient for contact dermatitis to heal. In order to use this criterion, either longer periods away from work or modification of the employee's job is generally necessary to allow the dermatitis time to resolve and the skin's barrier time for repair.

Criterion 7. Patch tests establish that an allergic contact dermatitis exists. Clinical relevance is established when it can be shown that the employee was exposed to that antigen at work. Patch testing should be performed according to standard procedures outlined in several texts concerning contact dermatitis.[2,9,13] Correct concentrations of antigens must be used in order to minimize false-positive or false-negative reactions. False-positive reactions may occur with the inappropriate use of irritating substances or as part of the excited skin syndrome.[7] False-negative patch test reactions occur when inappropriately low concentrations of test substances are used, when inappropriate vehicles for patch test substances are used, and when the patient is being treated with insufficiently high dosages of systemic steroids.

Preexisting Conditions

Workers' compensation laws also allow an employee to be compensated because the workplace caused a substantial aggravation of a preexisting dermatitis. When there is a reasonable probability that the dermatitis was aggravated by the job, the employee is compensable until the dermatitis has completely reverted to its clinical status before it was aggravated. Determining that the dermatitis is clinically more severe is aided subjectively by the patient's historical need to use more medication in the involved areas or objectively by the examiner's comparison with a previous clinical examination, if available. The spread of the preexisting dermatitis to previously uninvolved skin sites favors work-related aggravation of the dermatitis.

CONCLUSION

Industrially related contact dermatitis presents as an irritant reaction, a contact allergy, or an urticarial dermatitis. A workman's contact dermatitis would be considered work related if it can be proved that the employee was exposed to the antigen or irritant in the workplace. In addition to causing dermatitis, environmental substances found in the workplace may aggravate occupational dermatitis. Repeated episodes of dermatitis burden the worker with disability and discomfort and the employer with expense and lost production. In order to prevent occupational hand dermatitis, exposure of the worker to allergens and irritants must be controlled. Various articles of protective clothing are available to shield the employee from those hazardous industrial materials that cannot be removed or replaced. Cooperation among employee, employer, and health team is necessary to reduce and minimize the occurrence of occupation-related contact dermatitis.

ACKNOWLEDGMENT

This chapter is reprinted with permission from Occupational Hand and Upper Extremity Injuries and Diseases, edited by Morton L. Kasdan, M.D., Philadelphia, Hanley & Belfus, Inc., 1991.

REFERENCES

1. Adams RD (ed): Occupational skin diseases. Occup Med State Art Rev 1:1–360, 1988.
2. Adams RM: Occupational Skin Disease. New York, Grune & Stratton, 1983, pp 1–477.

3. Adams RM, Daily AD, Brancaccio RR, et al: Alstroemeria: A new and potent allergen for florists. Dermatol Clin 8:73–76, 1990.
4. Adams RM, Fisher AA: Contact allergen alternatives: 1986. J Am Acad Dermatol 14:951–969, 1986.
5. Berkley SF, Hightower AW, Beier RD, et al: Dermatitis in grocery workers associated with high natural concentrations of furanocoumarins in celery. Ann Intern Med 105:351–355, 1986.
6. Birmingham D: Occupational dermatology. In Demis DJ (ed): Clinical Dermatology. Philadelphia, J.B. Lippincott, 1989, pp 1–25.
7. Bruynzeel DP, Maibach HI: Excited skin syndrome (angry back). Arch Dermatol 122:323–328, 1986.
8. Cardullo AC, Ruszkowski AM, DeLeo VA: Allergic contact dermatitis resulting from sensitivity to citrus peel, geraniol, and citral. J Am Acad Dermatol 21:395–397, 1989.
9. Cronin E: Contact Dermatitis. Edinburgh, Churchill Livingstone, 1980, pp 1–915.
10. Cronin E: Clinical patterns of hand eczema in women. Contact dermatitis 13:153–161, 1985.
11. Dooms-Goossens AE, Debusschere KM, Gevers DM, et al: Contact dermatitis caused by airborne agents. J Am Acad Dermatol 15:1–10, 1986.
12. Edman B: Sites of contact dermatitis in relationship to particular allergens. Contact Dermatitis 13:129–135, 1985.
13. Fisher AA: Contact Dermatitis, 3rd ed. Philadelphia, Lea & Febiger, 1986, pp 1–954.
14. Fisher AA: Management of hairdressers sensitized to hair dyes or permanent wave solutions. Cutis 43:316–318, 1989.
15. Foussereau J, Tomb R, Cavelier C: Allergic contact dermatitis from safety clothes and individual protective devices. Dermatol Clin 8:127–132, 1990.
16. Heacock HJ, Rivers JK: Occupational diseases of hairdressers. Can J Public Health 77:109–113, 1986.
17. Herzog J, Dunne J, Aber R, et al: Milk tester's dermatitis. J Am Acad Dermatol 19:503–508, 1988.
18. Holness DL, Nethercott JR: Dermatitis in hairdressers. Dermatol Clin 8:119–126, 1990.
19. Kellet JK, Beck MH: Ammonium persulphate sensitivity in hairdressers. Contact Dermatitis 13:26–28, 1985.
20. Kligman AM: The spectrum of contact urticaria. Dermatol Clin 8:61–66, 1990.
21. Lammintausta K, Kalimo K: Atopy and hand dermatitis in hospital wet work. Contact Dermatitis 7:301–308, 1981.
22. Marks JG: Allergic contact dermatitis to *Alstroemeria.* Arch Dermatol 124:914–916, 1988.
23. Mathias CGT: Occupational dermatoses. J Am Acad Dermatol 19:1107–1114, 1988.
24. Mathias CGT: Contact dermatitis and workers' compensation: Criteria for establishing occupational causation and aggravation. J Am Acad Dermatol 20:842–848, 1989.
25. Mathias CGT, Morrison JH: Occupational skin disease, United States: Results from the Bureau of Labor Statistics annual survey of occupational injuries and illnesses, 1973 through 1984. Arch dermatol 124:1519–1524, 1988.
26. Menz J, Winkelmann RK: Sensitivity to wild vegetation. Contact Dermatitis 16:169–173, 1987.
27. Morrison LH, Storrs FJ: Persistence of an allergen in hair after glyceryl monothioglycolate-containing permanent wave solutions. J Am Acad Dermatol 19:52–59, 1988.
28. Moursiden HT, Faber O: Penetration of protective gloves by allergens and irritants. Trans St John's Hosp Dermatol Soc 59:230–234, 1973.
29. Nethercott JR, Holmes DC: Occupational dermatitis in food handlers and bakers. J Am Acad Dermatol 21:485–488, 1989.
30. Nethercott JR, MacPherson M, Choi BCK, Nixon P: Contact dermatitis in hairdressers. Contact Dermatitis 14:73–79, 1986.
31. Nilsson E, Mikaelsson B, Andersson S: Atopy, occupational and domestic work as risk factors for hand eczema in hospital workers. Contact Dermatitis 13:216–223, 1985.
32. Orchard S: Barrier creams. Dermatol Clin 2:616–629, 1984.
33. Reiss F, Fisher AA: Is hair dyed with para-phenylenediamine allergic? Arch Dermatol 109:221–222, 1974.
34. Rycroft RJG: Low humidity dermatoses. Dermatol Clin 2:553–559, 1984.
35. Schuman SH, Dobson RL: An outbreak of contact dermatitis in farm workers. J Am Acad Dermatol 13:220–223, 1985.
36. Storrs FJ: Permanent wave contact dermatitis: Contact allergy to glyceryl monothioglycolate. J Am Acad Dermatol 11:74–85, 1984.
37. Storrs FJ, Rosenthal LE, Adams RM, et al: Prevalence and relevance of allergic reactions in patients patch tested in North America—1984 to 1985. J Am Acad Dermatol 20:1038–1045, 1989.
38. Taylor JS: Allergic reaction to latex can be life-threatening. Skin Allergy News 20:2, 1989.

39. Taylor JS, Parrish JA, Blank IH: Environmental reactions to chemical, physical, and biologic agents. J Am Acad Dermatol 11:1007–1021, 1984.
40. Thiboutot DM, Hamory BH, Marks JG Jr: Dematoses among floral shop workers. J Am Acad Dermatol 22:54–58, 1990.
41. von Krogh G, Maibach HI: The contact urticaria syndrome—An updated review. J Am Acad Dermatol 5:328–342, 1981.
42. Warshawshki L, Mitchell JC, Storrs FJ: Allergic contact dermatitis from glyceryl monothioglycolate in hairdressers. Contact Dermatitis 7:351–352, 1981.
43. Weary PE: Prevention of skin disease. J Am Acad Dermatol 11:1022–1024, 1984.

BRIAN G. FORRESTER, MD, MPH

RUBBER CONTACT URTICARIA

Occupational Medicine Fellow
School of Hygiene and Public Health
Johns Hopkins University
Baltimore, Maryland

Reprint requests to:
Brian G. Forrester, MD, MPH
University of Alabama at Birmingham
Division of Occupational and Environmental Medicine
Birmingham, Alabama

Contact urticaria, characterized by the typical "wheal and flare" reaction of the skin, is a common reaction of the dermis to rapidly absorbed agents in the environment. The contact urticaria syndrome includes contact urticaria, as well as extracutaneous reactions such as anaphylaxis and asthma.[25] Rubber contact urticaria (RCU) refers to the induction of the symptoms of contact urticaria after exposure to allergens derived from natural latex.

Contact urticaria may be divided into the nonimmunologic, immunologic, and uncertain types.[10,25] Nonimmunologic contact urticaria is the most common type, occurs without prior sensitization, and is not antibody mediated.[10] The agents causing nonimmunologic contact urticaria may act through either one of two mechanisms: either as a direct influence on dermal vessel walls or as a result of the non-antibody-mediated release of vasoactive substances such as histamine, slow-reacting substance of anaphylaxis, or bradykinin.[9]

IDENTIFICATION

Immunologic contact urticaria differs from nonimmunologic contact urticaria in that it involves prior exposure to a sensitizing agent and is antibody mediated through the immediate release of immunoglobulin E (IgE).[25] Immunologic contact urticaria is the most common cause of occupationally related contact urticaria.

Contact urticaria has been a recognized phenomenon since the nineteenth century.[11] However, it was not until 1979 that Nutter described the first reported case of rubber contact urticaria, which was in a housewife who used rubber cleaning gloves for hand protection during housework.[14] One year later, Forstrom described the first case of occupationally related RCU, in a female nurse exposed to latex surgical gloves.[6] Since that time, more than 100 cases have been reported in the literature,[3] making this entity a recognized occupationally related disease that must be diagnostically considered in any case of contact urticaria.

In support of the theory that RCU is immunologic in origin, contact urticaria to rubber gloves appears to be IgE mediated. Frosch[7] and Turjanmaa and Reunala[23] have detected specific IgE antibodies to latex by radioimmunoassay in serum obtained from patients with RCU. Cell-mediated immune reactions do not appear to be of importance in immediate allergy to latex.[21]

The allergen that is presumed to be responsible for RCU is derived from the rubber tree, *Hevea brasiliensis,*[24] the source of latex for most latex products available in the marketplace.[2] Latex obtained from *H. brasiliensis* contains proteins, lipids, amino acids, nucleotides, and cofactors.[16] The final latex product obtained from *H. brasiliensis* contains approximately 2–3% protein.[16] The allergen that is thought to be responsible for RCU has been isolated by Carillo and associates and is a trypsin-sensitive protein with a molecular weight greater than 30,000 daltons.[4]

The lack of recognition of RCU prior to 1979 presents the question of whether this is a new condition with increasing incidence or whether it had simply gone unrecognized in the past. The recent increase in reporting of RCU may be due to one of three possibilities[3]: (1) The incidence is increasing due to more frequent use of latex gloves by health care workers in response to growing concerns over infectious disease. (2) RCU has been essentially unrecognized in the past. (3) Due to increasing worldwide demand for latex products, the latex manufacturing process has been altered in such a way that today's products more easily leach allergens from rubber gloves, causing the worker greater exposure now than previously. Factors influencing the release of contact urticaria allergens from latex products include duration of use, amount of close skin contact, and the effect of sweat.[20]

The allergenicity of the protein responsible for RCU appears to be more important than the total amount of protein eluting from a latex product.[20] The manufacturing process determines to a large extent whether the allergens that cause RCU are present in latex products. In a study of patients known to have RCU, Turjanmaa et al. found that gloves from 19 different manufacturers varied widely in their ability to produce positive skin prick tests (SPTs) in different patients.[20] Responses of the 19 different gloves tested ranged from a low of 8% positive SPTs to a high of 100% positive SPTs in the patients tested, demonstrating that the manufacturing process has a large impact on the allergenicity of the latex proteins present in different latex gloves. The same study performed high-pressure liquid chromatography tests on two of the latex gloves and found that the protein profiles were similar to that of natural rubber, indicating that proteins derived from natural rubber are able to survive the manufacturing process.

CAUSES

Sources of latex exposure that may cause RCU include latex gloves, balloons, dental cofferdams, rubber nipples, and latex condoms.[1,22] Similar to latex gloves, different brands of latex condoms appear to vary in their ability to induce urticarial reactions.[22] In addition, cross-reactivity exists between latex-glove-associated urticaria and latex-condom-associated urticaria, with one study reporting that 24% of patients known to have latex-glove-associated urticaria had experienced localized swelling and/or pruritus during intercourse using latex condoms.[22] This indicates that immunologically similar allergens are present in both latex gloves and latex condoms.

Risk factors that have been identified as important for the development of RCU include a history of atopic disease, preexisting hand eczema, exposure to latex gloves as a health care worker or during cleaning work, and chronic medical conditions requiring frequent exposure to latex products, such as spina bifida or multiple congenital urologic abnormalities.[17,23,26]

The most important risk factor for the development of RCU may be the lack of a functioning protective skin barrier, usually due to atopy or other dermatitides.[3] In one study, 67% of health care workers with RCU were atopics.[19] In eczema, the loss of the protective barrier function of the skin is thought to allow greater penetration of the latex allergen, thus resulting in greater exposure so that sensitization takes place more easily.

Patients with chronic debilitating medical conditions requiring frequent contact with rubber products, such as daily urinary bladder catheterizations or fecal disimpactions, also appear to have an increased risk of developing RCU.[17] Severe anaphylactic reactions during surgery have been reported in such patients.[17]

Undiagnosed persons with RCU are at serious risk if they are examined or operated on by medical personnel wearing latex surgical gloves.[23] Mucosal exposures may be particularly prone to result in anaphylactic reactions.[18] Anaphylactic reactions to latex have been reported during gynecologic examinations, dental examinations, surgery, and sexual intercourse using condoms.[1,2,18,26]

Possible sources of rubber exposure during surgery and anesthesia include latex surgical gloves, breathing bags, compressive bandages, and pharmaceuticals contaminated from rubber stoppers present on medication vials.[16] In one yearlong study by Leynadier et al., the authors found that 10% of all patients referred to their clinic for anaphylaxis occurring during surgery were due to rubber anaphylaxis (5 out of 43 cases).[12] Other types of allergic responses that may occur as part of the RCU syndrome include rhinitis, asthma, and angioedema.[4,13,15]

The association between health care workers and RCU is of special interest. In recent years, the increasing concern about the risk of contracting a blood-borne infectious disease has caused most health care workers to use latex gloves much of the time that they come in contact with patients, sometimes for as long as several hours a day. This increased usage of latex gloves has also increased the exposure of health care workers to the latex allergen. As mentioned previously, the increasing worldwide demand for latex gloves may have also resulted in manufacturing changes that increased the leachability of the latex allergen responsible for RCU. The result of these recent developments is that the frequency of occurrence of RCU is remarkably high.

In a prevalence study of RCU in health care providers, 7.4% of physicians and 5.6% of nurses working in operating units were found to have RCU.[19] This was significantly greater than prevalences found in non–health care workers ($p < .01$). In addition, an exposure gradient was found, with physicians and nurses in operating units having a significantly higher prevalence than those working in examination units or laboratories ($p < .01$).

TESTING AND DIAGNOSIS

The diagnosis of RCU is difficult to make by history and physical examination alone because most patients are clinically normal at the time of the examination, and the clinical history is often not helpful in establishing a diagnosis. Many patients present with nonspecific complaints such as itching, burning, or a history of recurrent hand eczema.[23] However, some patients do give diagnostically helpful histories of redness and wheal and flare reactions at the site of rubber contact. Their symptoms occur within minutes of contact with rubber and gradually subside over 1–2 hours if exposure is terminated.[23] The diagnosis is usually confirmed by provocation testing through epicutaneous means, by serology, or by in vitro confirmation. Methods of skin testing used to diagnose RCU include scratch chamber testing, SPT, and the whole-glove-use test.[23]

Scratch chamber testing may be performed by placing moistened glove pieces over scratches made on the volar forearm and covering with a Finn chamber.[23] Results are then graded based on the urticarial response. However, the scratch chamber test tends to give more false-positive responses than the SPT and delivers larger amounts of allergen to the patient, because it cannot be serially diluted. This increases the risk of potentially serious adverse reactions. Therefore, the scratch chamber test is considered by most investigators to be inferior to the SPT and is not recommended.

The SPT is more specific than the scratch chamber test and has fewer adverse reactions than the whole-glove-use test. Latex glove allergen for use in skin prick testing may be obtained by incubating 1 cm^2 strips of freshly cut latex gloves in 5 cc of sterile saline.[24] One drop of this solution is placed on the volar forearm, and the skin is lightly pricked with a small-gauge needle. Physiologic saline and histamine (10 mg/cc) may be used as controls. Reaction to SPT may be graded as 2+ when it is half the reaction to histamine, 3+ when it is equal to the histamine reaction, and 4+ when it is greater than the histamine reaction.[24] SPT is the diagnostic method of choice in most patients due to its ease in administration, rapid results, good patient tolerance, and low risk of adverse reactions.

The latex-glove-use test involves wearing the glove felt to be responsible for the urticarial reaction in an attempt to reproduce the typical urticarial response. It also gives good results, although it has a higher risk of adverse reactions than the SPT. It is recommended that the latex-glove-use test expose only one finger initially, in order to reduce the possibility of an anaphylactic reaction.[2] A whole glove should be worn only if the one-finger test is negative.

Latex-glove-use tests may be graded as 1+ if some redness occurs in the contact area, 2+ if fewer than 10 wheals are observed, and 3+ if 10 or more wheals are observed.[24] Contact should be maintained between the glove and the wet skin for at least 15 minutes. Contact durations lasting longer than 15 minutes are preferred because they give fewer false-negative results.[24]

In vitro diagnostic testing has also been used in the diagnosis of RCU, including the radioallergosorbent test (RAST) and the basophil histamine release test (BHRT). The latex RAST is a good indicator in highly allergic persons, but in those with mild allergy, the RAST does not appear to be as specific as the SPT or the latex-glove-use test.[24] It is also much more expensive, with a longer time interval present before results are known to the clinician.

The BHRT is a relatively new test that is promising to be useful in the diagnosis of rubber contact allergy. Methods for performing the test have been described by Turjanmaa et al., who found that in diagnosis of RCU, the BHRT was comparable to both the SPT and the latex-glove-use test and superior to the RAST.[21] The BHRT suffers, however, from limited availability, increased expense, and a longer time interval for diagnosis when compared with epicutaneous testing.

PREVENTION

Prevention of RCU requires substitution of a nonallergenic alternative. Persons performing nonsurgical or cleaning work may easily switch to vinyl gloves, which have very few allergic-related problems.[5] However, care should be taken when substituting vinyl for latex gloves to ensure that adequate protection against infectious agents is afforded. In a study comparing the quality and viral permeability of vinyl and latex gloves, Kotilainen et al. have shown that vinyl gloves tend to fail the watertightness test significantly more frequently than latex gloves (average 11.1% vs. 1.4%, $p < .001$).[8] Different brands of vinyl gloves also varied considerably in the proportion failing the watertightness test, ranging from 4% to 28%. In addition, unused, untested vinyl gloves demonstrated a 2.5–10% penetration of herpes simplex virus 1 (HSV-1) in laboratory testing. This penetration decreased significantly, to .95%, if the vinyl gloves were proved to be watertight beforehand. Vinyl gloves appear to be just as effective in preventing penetration of HSV-1 as latex gloves if they are proved to be intact, but the manufacturing process for vinyl gloves appears to allow a much higher percentage of defective gloves to reach the marketplace than is the case with latex gloves.

Substitution of vinyl gloves for latex is not possible for surgeons or nurses involved in operating rooms or emergency care. However, latex-allergic surgeons and nurses appear to be able to successfully circumvent their occupational allergy by switching glove brands or wearing undergloves. It appears to be quite rare that doctors or nurses use sick leave or switch professions due to RCU.[19]

In summary, RCU is an important cause of occupational contact urticaria and appears to be increasing in frequency. Persons at risk of developing RCU include health care workers, cleaning workers, persons with atopia or other dermatitides, and patients with chronic medical conditions requiring frequent exposure to latex products. RCU may also include other systemic reactions, such as rhinitis, asthma, angioedema, and anaphylaxis. Confirming the diagnosis of RCU requires epicutaneous or in vitro testing, with skin prick testing as the diagnostic method of choice. Prevention of RCU may be accomplished in some workers by product substitution. Latex-sensitized workers may benefit by switching glove brands or wearing undergloves.

REFERENCES

1. Axelsson IGK, Eriksson M, Wrangsjö K, et al: Anaphylaxis and angioedema due to rubber allergy in children. Acta Paediatr Scand 77:314–316, 1988.
2. Axelsson JGK, Johansson SGO, Wrangsjö K, et al: IgE mediated anaphylactoid reactions to rubber. Allergy 42:46–50, 1987.
3. Belsito DV: Contact urticaria caused by rubber. Analysis of seven cases. Dermatol Clin 8(1):61–66, 1990.
4. Carrillo T, Cuevas M, Munoz T, et al: Contact urticaria and rhinitis from latex surgical gloves. Contact Dermatitis 15:69–72, 1986.
5. Estlander T, Jolanki R, Kanerra L, et al: Dermatitis and urticaria from rubber and plastic gloves. Contact Dermatitis 14:20–25, 1986.
6. Forstrom L: Contact urticaria from latex surgical gloves. Contact Dermatitis 6:33–34, 1980.
7. Frosch PJ, Wahl R, Bahmer FA, et al: Contact urticaria to rubber gloves is IgE mediated. Contact Dermatitis 14:241–245, 1986.
8. Kotilainen HR, Brinker JP, Avato JL, et al: Latex and vinyl examination gloves: Quality control procedures and implications for health care workers. Arch Intern Med 149:2749–2753, 1989.
9. Lahti A: Non-immunologic contact urticaria. Acta Derm Venereol 60(Suppl 91):3–49, 1980.
10. Lahti A, Maibach HI: Immediate contact reactions (contact urticaria syndrome). In Maibach HI (ed): Occupational and Industrial Dermatology. Chicago, Year Book, 1987, pp 32–44.

11. Lesser E: Lehrbuch der Haut—und Geschlechtskrankheiten für studirende und ärzte. Capitel: Urticaria. Leipzig, Verlag von F.C.W. Vogel, 1894, p 134.
12. Leynadier F, Pecquet C, Dry J, et al: Anaphylaxis to latex during surgery. Anaesthesia 44:547–550, 1989.
13. Lozynsky OA, Dupuis L, Shandling B, et al: Anaphylactoid and systemic reactions following saline enema administration. Ann Allergy 56:62–66, 1986.
14. Nutter AF: Contact urticaria to rubber. Br J Dermatol 101:597–598, 1979.
15. Seaton A, Cherrie B, Turnbull J, et al: Rubber glove asthma. BMJ 296:531–532, 1988.
16. Slater JE: Rubber anaphylaxis. N Engl J Med 320:1126–1130, 1989.
17. Swartz J, Braude BM, Gilmour RR, et al: Intraoperative anaphylaxis to latex. Can J Anaesth 37:589–592, 1990.
18. Taylor JS, Cassettari J, Wagner W, et al: Contact urticaria and anaphylaxis to latex. J Am Acad Dermatol 21:874–877, 1989.
19. Turjanmaa K: Incidence of immediate allergy to latex gloves in hospital personnel. Contact Dermatitis 17:270–275, 1987.
20. Turjanmaa K, Laurila K, Mäkinen-Kiljunen S, et al: Rubber contact urticaria allergenic properties of 19 brands of latex gloves. Contact Dermatitis 19:362–367, 1988.
21. Turjanmaa K, Rasanen L, Lehto M, et al: Basophil histamine release and lymphocyte proliferation tests in latex contact urticaria. Allergy 44:181–186, 1989.
22. Turjanmaa K, Reunala T: Condoms as a source of latex allergen and cause of contact urticaria. Contact Dermatitis 20:360–364, 1989.
23. Turjanmaa K, Reunala T: Contact urticaria from rubber gloves. Dermatol Clin 6(1):47–51, 1988.
24. Turjanmaa K, Reunala T, Räsänen L, et al: Comparison of diagnostic methods in latex surgical glove contact urticaria. Contact Dermatitis 19:241–247, 1988.
25. Von Krogh G, Maibach HI: Contact urticaria. In Adams RM (ed): Occupational Skin Disease. New York, Grune & Stratton, 1983, pp 58–69.
26. Zenarola P: Rubber latex allergy: Unusual complication during surgery. Contact Dermatitis 21:197–198, 1989.

NIELS K. VEIEN, MD, PHD

NICKEL SENSITIVITY AND OCCUPATIONAL SKIN DISEASE

From The Dermatology Clinic
Vesterbro 99
DK-9000 Aalborg, Denmark

Reprint requests to:
Niels K. Veien, MD, PhD
The Dermatology Clinic
Vesterbro 99
DK-9000 Aalborg, Denmark

Dermatologists who engage in patch testing identify nickel as the most frequently occurring contact allergen. When, at the same time, we consider that nickel is one of the most common metals in the crust of the earth, we see why this allergen is of such interest for physicians engaged in the treatment and prevention of occupational skin diseases.

Nickel is a shiny, silvery, corrosion-resistant metal. It is mined in Canada, Russia, and several other countries and can be produced at relatively low cost. It is widely used in industry in various alloys and is used extensively to plate other metals.

Nickel is present in fossil fuels such as coal. It is also found in fertilizers and sewage sludge. The environmental load is therefore likely to increase in industrial areas.[21,53]

Nickel is an essential element for several species of laboratory animals, but it has not as yet been proved that it is an essential element for humans.[41] In large doses, inorganic nickel salts can be toxic. The routes of human exposure to nickel include the gastrointestinal tract, the respiratory system, and the skin.

One serious health hazard associated with nickel is the carcinogenic potential of some nickel salts, notably the highly toxic nickel carbonyl, in the upper respiratory tract, in particular, the nose.[30,66] A few reports indicate that immediate-type hypersensitivity to nickel may lead to asthma and allergic rhinitis.[4,45] That type of reaction is probably rare.

Quantitatively, the primary health hazard associated with nickel is delayed-type sensitization to nickel, resulting in allergic contact dermatitis.

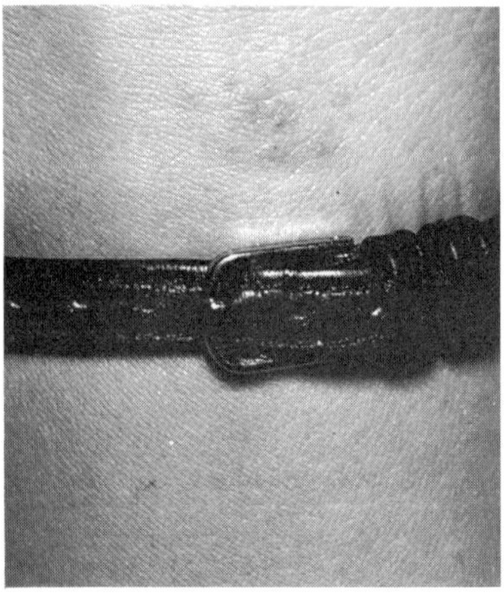

FIGURE 1. Allergic nickel contact dermatitis from a nickel-plated watch strap buckle.

SENSITIZATION

Nickel ions readily penetrate the skin. Sensitization takes place after nickel is presented to the immune system by the Langerhans cells. Nickel-specific T cells are presumably produced in the paracortical areas of the regional lymph nodes. These T cells circulate, and once one has become sensitized to nickel, even in a small area of the body (Fig. 1), one will react to the metal wherever it makes contact with the skin surface.

The diagnostic test that is used to demonstrate nickel sensitivity in vivo is occluded patch testing with 5% nickel sulfate. The test is best read after 72 hours (Fig. 2). Because of the many pitfalls inherent in patch testing, the procedure should be carried out by a trained dermatologist with experience in performing it.

Nickel salts do not readily sensitize laboratory animals, and under experimental conditions, nickel is not considered to be a strong allergen in humans.[58,67] This

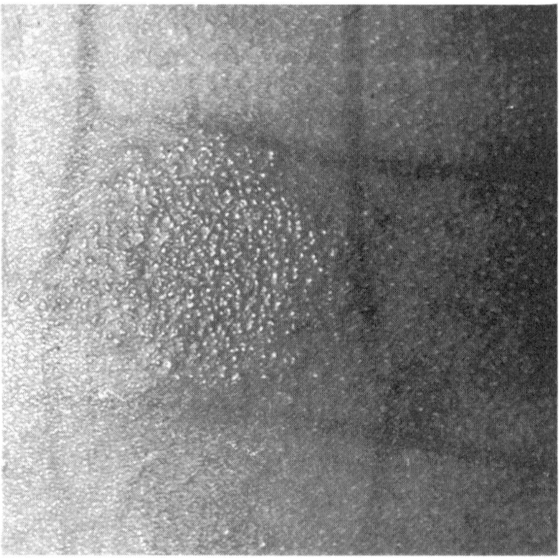

FIGURE 2. A positive patch test to 5% nickel sulfate in petrolatum after 48 hours.

TABLE 1. Number of Positive Patch Tests to Nickel in Some Major Patch Test Studies

Authors and Type of Study	Period of the Study	No. Tested (% with positive patch tests to nickel)	
		Men	Women
Nethercott et al., multicenter[43]	Aug. 1985–July 1989	2,012 (5.8)	2,928 (16.1)
Enders et al., one clinic[13]	1977–83 inclusive	4,775 (2.6)	7,202 (13.7)
Gola et al., multicenter[19]	1984–88 inclusive	23,541 (31%)	
Christophersen et al., multicenter[6]	Sept. 1985–Feb 1986	696 (5.1)	1,470 (20.7)

information contrasts with the fact that patch test studies carried out in many countries indicate that contact sensitization to nickel is very common. The results of a few of the major studies are given in Table 1. It can be seen that whereas 10–30% of the women tested in these studies had positive nickel patch tests, only a small percentage of the men tested positive.

Prevalence studies carried out by Menné in the early 1980s indicated that, at that time, 1% of Danish men and 10% of Danish women were sensitive to nickel.[32]

The rate of nickel sensitization is increasing in most countries. Studies carried out over long periods of time and involving large numbers of patients are listed in Table 2.

In 1991, a statutory order was implemented in Denmark prohibiting the use of nickel-plated items intended for close contact with the skin, such as buttons, belt buckles, watch strap buckles, eyeglass frames, and jewelry.[2,35] The order stipulates that the amount of nickel released from the listed items must be less than 0.5 $\mu g/cm^2$/week. A dimethylglyoxime test (described later) should be negative. As this statutory order takes effect, the incidence of nickel sensitization in Denmark should decrease.

TABLE 2. Patch Testing with Nickel: A Comparison of Results Obtained during Two Different Periods

Authors and Type of Study	Total No. of Persons Patch Tested and Period Covered	No. of Positive Patch Tests to Nickel (% positive)			
Gola et al., multicenter[19]	23,541 (1984–88)			1984	1988
		Nonoccupational		934 (23.8)	1452 (45.5)
		Occupational allergic contact dermatitis		181 (13.0)	218 (18.2)
Vcien et al., one clinic[56]	10,423 (1975–80) and (1986–90)	1975–80		1986–90	
		Men	Women	Men	Women
		55 (4.2)	411 (15.5)	64 (2.9)	706 (17.4)
Gollhausen et al., one clinic[20]	11,962 (1977–82)	1977		1982	
		Men	Women	Men	Women
	Estimated	(1.5)	(10.5)	(3.8)	(15)
Edman & Möller, one clinic[10]	8,933 (1969–80)	1969		1980	
	Estimated	(1)	(11)	(1.5)	(18)

When nickel dermatitis was first described, most of those sensitized were men employed in the galvanizing industry. At that time, nickel dermatitis was thought of as a predominantly occupational problem. Although today most sensitizations occur among women (Tables 1 and 2), men in the galvanizing industries may still be at risk.[63] Some authors have speculated that there is a sex-related difference in the tendency to become sensitized to nickel, but no substantial evidence for such a difference has been discovered to date. It is generally accepted that differences in exposure patterns provide the best explanation for the sex-related difference.

Studies carried out in Sweden in recent years indicate that the popular practice of piercing the ears of both men and women is a major cause of nickel sensitization (Fig. 3). Larsson-Stymne's and Widström's[29] examination of 960 schoolgirls showed that 72% of the girls had pierced ears. Twenty of 126 8-year-olds (16%) with pierced ears had nickel allergy, compared with 2 of 159 girls (1%) who did not have pierced ears. Forty-three of 335 15-year-old girls (13%) with pierced ears had nickel allergy compared with 0 of 36 girls (0%) who did not have pierced ears. Curiously, the rate of nickel sensitization among girls who have their ears pierced is much higher than the rate among men with pierced ears.[64]

Nickel sensitization usually takes place at a young age, and most girls become sensitized during their teens.[13,55] The fact that sensitization commonly occurs before these young women are engaged in an occupation complicates the evaluation of the occupational relationship of nickel contact dermatitis. Today occupational nickel dermatitis is typically an elicitation of nickel dermatitis in an already sensitized person.

Sensitivity to nickel is persistent. All of 100 patients with positive patch tests to nickel reacted to the metal when retested 10 years later.[26]

Nickel sensitivity in women is often associated with cobalt allergy, and it has been debated whether simultaneous sensitization occurs due to the concomitant presence of nickel and cobalt in many alloys. An adjuvant mechanism has been suggested in laboratory animals.[28] It has also been argued that cobalt allergy is a

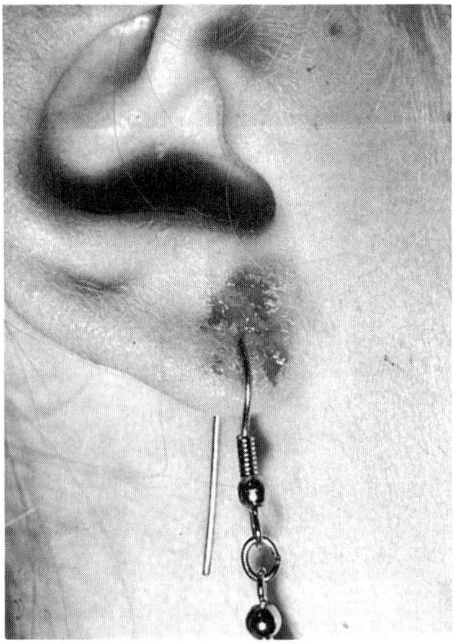

FIGURE 3. Allergic nickel contact dermatitis associated with ear piercing.

secondary sensitization. The concomitant sensitization is often related to persistent hand eczema.[33,52]

OCCURRENCE

Nickel and nickel salts are used as follows.

Electroplating

Nickel-plated items have shiny surfaces that are virtually noncorrosive. The nickel coating has little mechanical strength, however, and a nickel-plated surface wears off easily. Nickel plating is, therefore, not suitable for faucets or similar, frequently used household items. Such items are usually chrome plated over a nickel undercoat. Nickel undercoating is also common with other types of metal plating such as gold plating. Nickel plating is used mainly in the manufacture of inexpensive jewelry, metal frames for eyeglasses, buttons, belt buckles, wristwatches, zippers, scissors, hairpins, kitchen utensils, suspender clasps, and the like.

Electronics

Semiconductors often contain nickel. Various electronic components may be nickel plated.

Pigments

Nickel salts can be used in ceramic paint and are also sometimes used in other types of paint.

Catalysts

Nickel powder mixed with other metals such as copper and aluminium is used as a catalyst to hydrogenate fats and thus change them from a liquid to a solid state.

Textiles

Nickel salts are used as mordants in dyeing textiles.

Nickel is used in a number of alloys as follows.

Stainless Steel

This alloy typically contains 10% nickel, 20% chromium, and 70% iron. The metals are so tightly bound in stainless steel that they are not easily released. Most nickel-sensitive persons tolerate contact with good-quality stainless steel, even when it is in close contact with the skin. Sweat and household detergents may release nickel from certain types of stainless steel in amounts sufficient to cause nickel contact dermatitis.[25]

Nickel Copper

This alloy, of 25% nickel and 75% copper, is widely used for coinage.

Nickel Chrome and Nickel Iron

These alloys are used in the aerospace and automotive industries.

Nickel Aluminium

This alloy is used in the manufacture of permanent magnets.

Nickel Cadmium

This alloy is used in the manufacture of rechargeable batteries.

White Gold

This alloy is composed of gold with approximately 15% nickel and may also contain palladium and silver. It is used for making jewelry.

Nickel Silver

This alloy contains 12% nickel, 24% zinc, and 64% copper. It is used for making jewelry.

In addition to the possible exposure to nickel by way of the aforementioned industrial and consumer products, some people are also occupationally exposed to nickel in areas of the world where it is mined. Cutaneous exposure may also come from detergents used for washing clothes or dishes, household and industrial cleansers, bleaching agents, and cosmetics.[1] The amount of nickel in such consumer products is so low, however, that it would not cause a flare-up of dermatitis even in most sensitized individuals. Basketter et al. have suggested that an amount of nickel of less than 5 ppm is an acceptable standard and that, ideally, the amount should be less than 1 ppm.[1] Pecegueiro found 22–45 ppm of nickel in one fertilizer,[46] and 5–10 ppm has been found in recycled paper used for toilet tissue.[3] Theoretically, that amount could cause perianal eczema in nickel-sensitive persons. Welding fumes and nickel in welding electrodes may cause flares of nickel dermatitis.[66]

Emmett et al. tested 12 nickel-sensitive patients with serial dilutions of nickel and found wide variations in the amounts of nickel in consumer products needed to cause a reaction in these patients.[12] The most sensitive patient reacted to 0.47 μg nickel; the least sensitive reacted to 5.2 mg. This study showed that, experimentally, synthetic sweat and plasma were more effective than saline in releasing nickel from metal objects.

Attempts have been made to produce alloys that may be safely used in making inexpensive jewelry. Romaguera et al. carried out a study of 964 patients with histories of metal intolerance and 200 controls with no known allergies.[49] All were patch tested with nickel sulfate and eight washers containing either nickel, nickel palladium, copper, brass, bronze, palladium, gold, or iron. Of the patients with histories of metal intolerance, 63% reacted to nickel sulfate, 50% reacted to the nickel washer, 8% to the nickel-palladium washer, 13% to the copper washer, 7% to the brass washer, 4% to the bronze or palladium washers, 2% to gold, and none to iron.

Menné et al.[34] studied the in vitro corrosion stability of 12 disks made of various metals and alloys and tested the patch test reactivity of nickel-sensitive patients to the same disks. They found that metals and alloys that release more than 1 μg nickel/cm^2/week in synthetic sweat gave strongly positive patch tests in nickel-sensitive patients, whereas metals that release less than 0.5 μg nickel/cm^2/week produced few positive patch tests. Stainless steel, white gold, and tin were considered "safe"; the nickel-tin alloy was found to be "relatively safe."

OCCUPATIONAL EXPOSURE

Persons in the workplace can be exposed to nickel in a number of occupations, including jobs in the electroplating industry and in the manufacture of the previously mentioned nickel alloys. A report on the evaluation of carcinogenic risks to humans from chromium, nickel, and welding presents a detailed review of the degree of nickel exposure in the nickel industry.[66]

There are a wide variety of nickel-plated items in many workplaces, including uniform buttons, hand tools, musical instruments, office equipment, and sewing equipment. Limited exposure to these items rarely causes nickel sensitization. However, already-nickel-sensitized employees in workplaces where there is cutaneous exposure to nickel salts and nickel alloys that release significant amounts of nickel risk the reactivation of their nickel dermatitis. This is also true in manufacturing jobs in which alloys and other substances that contain nickel are used—typically the manufacture of metal items. Exposure may occur from contact with the metals themselves or with metal dust during the manufacturing process or when nickel is leached from the metals into cutting fluids. This last form of exposure does not appear to be a major cause of reactivation of nickel dermatitis.[11]

Frequent handling of coins caused fingertip dermatitis in a shop assistant. The dermatitis appeared mostly on the fingers of the right hand—the hand used to collect the coins (Fig. 4).

Ceramic workers engaged as decorators had a high prevalence of nickel sensitivity (20 of 64 workers, or 31.2%) compared with those who worked as enamelers (8 of 126, or 6.3%).[40] A list of occupations in which there is exposure to nickel is given in Table 3.

More curious examples of occupational nickel contact dermatitis include cases seen on the necks of physicians and nurses who wear stethoscopes around the neck. A teacher developed hand dermatitis from chalk that by means of the dimethylglyoxime test was shown to contain nickel.[48] A male butcher developed dermatitis due to a nickel-plated button in his protective steel glove (Fig. 5). One worker developed dermatitis after flame spraying with metals.[22] This author has seen nickel dermatitis caused by the plastic cabinet used to hold a cordless telephone. The plastic cabinet contained nickel.

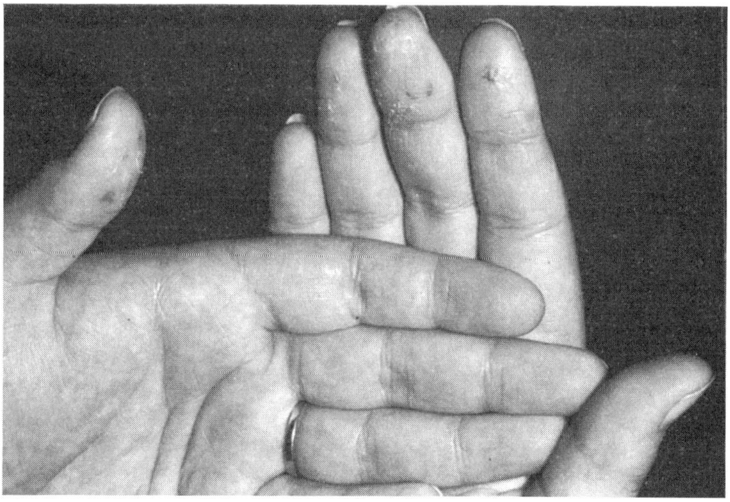

FIGURE 4. Occupational allergic contact dermatitis on fingertips intensively exposed to coins containing nickel. Note dermatitis on the tips of the 2nd, 3rd, and 4th fingers of the right hand and the left thumb.

TABLE 3. Typical Occupations with Nickel Exposure

Auto mechanic	Enameler
Cashier	Hairdresser
Ceramic worker	Jeweler
Cleaner	Metalworker
Construction worker	Printing industry worker
Dentist and dental assistant	Production line worker
Electronics industry worker	Radio and TV repair person
Electroplater	

Increased amounts of nickel may also be released from metallic objects due to sweating, high temperatures, pressure, and the acidic substances in hairdressing liquids and some foods.[14,23,36]

Those employed in specific occupations that entail significant nickel exposure risk nickel sensitization, but nickel dermatitis is also often seen in those who have traditionally "wet" occupations such as cleaning, nursing, hairdressing, housekeeping, and food preparation. Such occupations may cause maceration of the skin of the hands, and the macerated skin is probably more easily penetrated by nickel than healthy skin is. In such cases, even a low concentration of nickel may cause dermatitis.

It is difficult to counsel a nickel-allergic person who has had to give up a job because of dermatitis. The best advice is probably a recommendation to choose a "dry" occupation in which one is not confronted with continuous exposure to nickel. Because much of the equipment in modern offices is made of plastic, office work can be suggested; teaching and caring for school-age children are also relatively dry jobs, as are selling jobs, except for the job of cashier.

CLINICAL FEATURES AND DIAGNOSIS

The diagnosis of occupational nickel dermatitis is easily made when a nickel-sensitive patient presents with a patch of dermatitis at a site that has been in obvious contact with a metal item used in the workplace and not during leisure time. This, however, is probably the least common of occupational problems

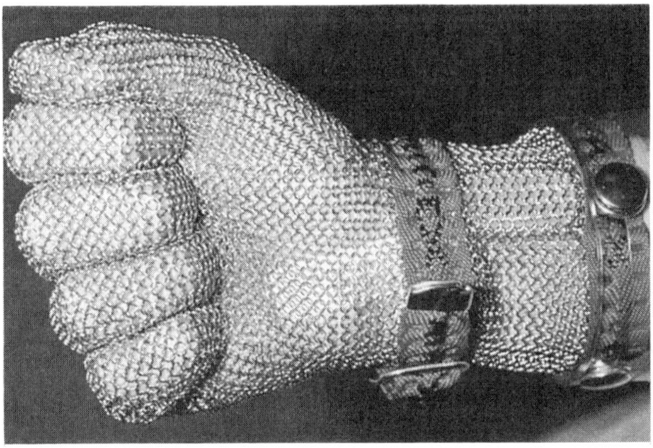

FIGURE 5. A butcher's protective steel glove, which caused occupational allergic contact dermatitis of the forearm where a nickel-plated button was in direct contact with the skin.

associated with nickel allergy. However difficult, it is therefore necessary to attempt to define the relationship between nickel and the workplace.

Nethercott et al. found that a worker was believed to have occupational dermatitis when it was established to have arisen "in the course of" and "out of" the worker's job.[44]

Rycroft defines occupational contact dermatitis as contact dermatitis due wholly or partially to the patient's occupation and adds that stricter definitions may be necessary for medicolegal questions of causations.[50]

The distinction between occupational and nonoccupational dermatitis is indeed difficult, as it also is when dealing with allergic contact dermatitis caused by nickel.

Generally speaking, 80–90% of patients with occupational skin disease present with hand dermatitis, perhaps in combination with dermatitis of the forearms. The relationship between hand eczema and nickel allergy is a complicated one, and the question of whether nickel-sensitive persons are more prone to develop hand eczema than non-nickel-sensitive persons has also been raised.

Since at least 10% of adult women have nickel allergy, and the prevalence of hand eczema among adult women is approximately 6%, a coincidence of nickel allergy and hand eczema will occur in women regardless of their occupation. Very few women are exposed to nickel solely in their professional life, and the primary irritants that induce or aggravate hand eczema are certainly factors in the lives of most women, whether they hold jobs outside the home or not.

Wilkinson and Wilkinson carefully reviewed the literature concerning the relationship between hand eczema and nickel allergy.[65] They discussed the morphology of hand eczema and found that there are few good studies dealing with the clinical features of hand eczema and its association with nickel allergy. The Wilkinsons present the following information:

a. A contact pattern of nickel dermatitis is uncommon, or rarely reported, because it is felt to be obvious. The authors state that, in their personal experience, a contact pattern on the hands caused by nickel items in a nickel-sensitive patient is unusual. This is also true for eczema on the dorsal aspects of the hands, usually considered to be caused by external contactants.
b. Palmar hyperkeratotic eczema gave a very low yield of positive patch tests to nickel.
c. Pompholyx (recurrent vesicular hand eczema), a hand eczema, associated with a number of often endogenous causes of eczema, is associated with nickel allergy. It has been debated whether or not this type of dermatitis is an example of systemically induced allergic contact dermatitis. It is the opinion of this author that the results of oral challenge studies and case reports of flares of vesicular hand eczema occurring after operations in which nickel alloy items are left in the body, for example, to assist in the healing of fractures, support such an association.
d. Hand eczema in nickel-sensitive patients is commonly of a nonspecific morphology, and the association between the nickel allergy and the hand eczema is uncertain. In specific occupations, particularly those involving wet work, the nickel allergy is probably partially relevant.

Wilkinson and Wilkinson conclude that there is a poorer prognosis for the hand eczema of those who also have nickel allergy than for those who do not, particularly if the former have dermatitis of a recurrent, vesicular morphology. Another factor that slows the improvement of hand eczema is the presence of more than one allergy. In adults, nickel allergy appears to aggravate the course of atopic dermatitis.[65]

Edman found a statistically significant correlation between nickel allergy and dermatitis on the palms, as well as the interdigital areas and dorsal aspects of the fingers.[9] Cronin, however, found no anatomical relationship between nickel allergy and hand dermatitis.[8]

The best criterion for a causative occupational factor is a definite occupational source of nickel exposure and the clearing of the hand eczema once that source has been removed. Other evidence suggesting an occupational cause of nickel dermatitis is the clearing of the dermatitis during vacations of three weeks' duration or more or during sick leave of the same length of time, followed by recurrence of the dermatitis upon resumption of work.

Once again, such clear associations are rare. It is more common to find nickel exposure both at work and in the home and to find some improvement of nickel dermatitis, but not clearing, when the patient is not at work and in turn aggravation upon resumption of work.

The complex relationship between nickel allergy and hand eczema suggests that there are several possible occupational relationships. The relationship may be definite, probable, or possible, or there may be no occupational relationship at all.

If the entire spectrum of occupational skin diseases—not only those associated with nickel allergy—is considered, then a category indicating occupational aggravation rather than occupational cause should also be added. This would apply, for example, in cases of hyperkeratotic palmar eczema aggravated by a person's occupation, as well as palmar psoriasis or lichen planus that is aggravated, but not caused by, the occupation of the patient.

The determination of whether or not a particular job and the nickel allergy of an individual patient are related is based on (1) a detailed knowledge of the risk of exposure to nickel, in combination with (2) an evaluation of the pattern of dermatitis, (3) the fluctuations of the dermatitis during prolonged absence from the workplace (usually more than one week) and upon the resumption of work, (4) an inspection of the workplace, and (5) a dimethylglyoxime test of the items suspected to cause or aggravate the dermatitis.

The dimethylglyoxime test is a spot test that consists of a 10% ammonium hydroxide solution and a 10% alcohol solution of dimethylglyoxime. A drop of each solution is absorbed into the cotton on a cotton-tipped applicator, which is then rubbed against the metal object for 30 seconds. A bright-red color on the metal object indicates the presence of nickel. The detection limit is approximately 0.5 μg nickel/cm^2.[60]

The determination of systemic occupational exposure to nickel in exposed individuals usually rests on the determination of nickel in urine and serum.[66]

Attempts have been made to determine the levels of occupational exposure to nickel by examining nail clippings. Peters et al. found high levels of nickel in the fingernails of persons employed in the electroplating industry.[47] Gammelgaard and Veien found higher levels of nickel in the nails of nickel-sensitive persons who had hand eczema than in the nails of nickel-sensitive persons with no hand eczema.[16]

Even though the occupational association between hand eczema and nickel allergy is difficult to prove for the individual patient, several studies of groups of patients provide circumstantial evidence indicating an association.

Fregert found nickel to be the most common allergen among 595 women with occupational dermatoses seen over a 10-year period.[15] The percentage of nickel-sensitive women increased from 9% to 19% during the study period. The majority of the nickel-sensitive women were in cleaning occupations or were hairdressers. In a follow-up study, the dermatitis of these nickel-sensitive women was found to have a poor prognosis.

Meding and Swanbeck found service work, most commonly cleaning, to have a significant association with occupational hand eczema.[31] The most common contact allergens seen in this study were nickel and cobalt.

In a joint study of 1,039 cases of occupational dermatoses studied by 27 dermatologists in a particular region of Denmark, nickel was by far the most common allergen affecting those with allergic contact dermatitis, particularly women. Most of the women concerned carried out wet work such as nursing, cleaning, and cooking.[57]

Clemmensen et al. found that the level of nickel in the water used for hospital cleaning increased throughout the course of the work day.[7]

Wall and Gebauer examined 993 persons with occupational skin diseases in Western Australia.[63] They found that 25% of 103 women whose occupational skin problem was allergic contact dermatitis had nickel allergy, which was considered relevant for their dermatitis. In a follow-up study, it was shown that more than 50% of the women had persistent symptoms of allergic contact dermatitis six months to eight years after the initial examination.[62]

Wall has shown that nickel penetrates rubber gloves, but not those made of polyvinyl chloride.[59] This is important information for those in occupations where there is extensive exposure to nickel.

One hundred and nineteen of 134 nickel-sensitive patients studied by Gawkrodger et al. were women.[17] Thirty-seven worked in offices, and 65 had occupations that included wet work.

Van der Burg et al. studied 303 student nurses and junior hairdressers.[5] There was a 26% prevalence of nickel allergy among the junior hairdressers, and the allergy had typically been acquired before the start of their training. Twelve percent of the student nurses had nickel allergy.

Nethercott and Holness examined 119 patients with nickel allergy, and an attempt was made to assess the relevance of the results obtained when these patients were patch tested.[42] The authors found no preponderance of nickel allergy among those engaged in particular occupations. In another, multicenter study involving 282 patients with work-related dermatoses, Nethercott et al. found no association between nickel allergy and particular jobs when these were compared with 1,250 persons who had nonoccupational dermatoses.[44]

Goh did not find a preponderance of nickel allergy among 217 cases of occupational hand eczema when these were compared with 504 cases of nonoccupational hand eczema.[18]

There is no definite link between nickel contact dermatitis and atopic dermatitis, and most studies suggest that persons with atopic dermatitis have an unchanged or slightly impaired propensity to develop contact sensitivity.[37]

A multivariate analysis carried out among 2,166 patch-tested patients showed that nickel allergy was significantly less common among atopics than among non-atopics.[6] Moorthy and Tan found a slightly higher prevalence of atopy among nickel-sensitive persons than among those with no nickel allergy.[39] Atopic persons with dermatitis persisting into adulthood had a higher number of contact sensitivities than those whose dermatitis had cleared. Nickel was among the common contact allergens in another study.[51] In yet another study, nickel sensitization tended to aggravate the course of the atopic dermatitis of adults, particularly hand dermatitits.[27]

Negative patch tests to nickel in patients with a history of nickel allergy were linked to atopy in one study,[38] while in another no such association was seen.[54]

PROGNOSIS

Allergic contact dermatitis caused by nickel and dichromate is notorious for a poor prognosis if the dermatitis is on the hands. Menné et al. found nickel allergy among 99 of 298 persons who had applied for permanent disability pensions in Denmark.[34] Most of these nickel-sensitive patients also had other sensitivities, typically to cobalt and/or dichromate.

PREVENTION

All available evidence indicates that extensive cutaneous contact with nickel-plated items is the cause of most sensitizations to nickel. In women, nonoccupational sensitization, usually from inexpensive metal earrings used after the ears have been pierced, is by far more common than occupational sensitization. In men, occupational sensitization occurs, but the problems associated with nickel allergy are less common in men than in women.

Once a person is sensitized to nickel, nickel dermatitis may be elicited by both nonoccupational and occupational sources, and the following discusses preventive measures.

1. In order to reduce exposure to sensitizing doses of nickel, particularly among young women, and to reduce the amounts of nickel handled in the workplace and during leisure time, legislation can be enacted. As of January 1, 1991, the sale of nickel-plated items intended for close contact with the skin has been prohibited in Denmark. Items such as zippers, buttons, belt buckles, watch strap buckles, frames for eyeglasses, hairpins, and earrings are covered by this ban. A maximum amount of 0.5 μg nickel/cm^2/week may be released from such items.[2,35] Items that prove negative when the dimethylglyoxime test is performed are considered safe. This intervention should lead to a reduction of the incidence of nickel sensitization in Denmark in years to come. Trivial eruptions of nickel dermatitis in already sensitized individuals caused by negligence in avoiding nickel in clothing and jewelry should also become less common after the introduction of this statutory code. Attempts are currently underway to introduce similar bans in the European Community.

2. A general reduction in the amounts of nickel available for penetration of the skin both in the workplace and outside it can be achieved through the use of metals and alloys from which there is a limited release of nickel. Stainless steel, tin, nickel tin, and white gold cause very few reactions in nickel-sensitive patients.[34]

3. For those who are already sensitized to nickel before they enter the workplace, it is important to provide preemployment counseling so as to prevent job choices that can lead to occupational nickel dermatitis. Jobs with obvious nickel contact should be avoided, and nickel-sensitive women should also avoid wet work.

4. Good skin care programs should be adopted in the workplace. If there are wet work and exposure to nickel, then vinyl gloves rather than rubber gloves should be worn because nickel may penetrate rubber gloves.[59]

5. Animal experiments and clinical studies suggest that it is possible to induce tolerance to nickel. In a study of young girls who had their ears pierced and also wore orthodontic braces, it was shown that if orthodontic treatment preceded ear piercing, significantly fewer girls would develop nickel allergy than if ear piercing preceded orthodontic treatment. Similarly, experiments with laboratory animals have shown that oral exposure to nickel prior to cutaneous contact with a sensitizing dose of nickel reduces the risk of sensitization.[24] These results may have some bearing on future attempts to prevent nickel sensitization.

REFERENCES

1. Basketter DA, Briatico-Vangosa G, Kaestner W, et al: Nickel, cobalt and chromium in consumer products: A role in allergic contact dermatitis? Contact Dermatitis 28:15–25, 1993.
2. Bekendtgørelse om forbud mod salg af visse nikkelholdige produkter [Statutory code prohibiting the sale of certain products containing nickel]. Miljøministeriets bekendtgørelse nr. 472 af 27. juni 1989 [Ministry of the Environment Statutory Code no. 472 of 27 June 1989]. Copenhagen, Ministry of the Environment, 1989.
3. Blecher P, Korting HC: Irritative und allergologische Aspekte der Verwendung Altpapier-haltiger Hygienepapiere im Analbereich. Derm Beruf Umwelt 40:30–34, 1992.
4. Block GT, Yeung M: Asthma induced by nickel. JAMA 247:1600–1602, 1982.
5. van der Burg CKH, Bruynzeel DP, Vreeburg KJJ, et al: Hand eczema in hairdressers and nurses: A prospective study. Contact Dermatitis 14:275–279, 1986.
6. Christophersen J, Menné T, Tanghøj P, et al: Clinical patch test data evaluated by multivariate analysis. Contact Dermatitis 21:291–299, 1989.
7. Clemmensen OJ, Menné T, Kaaber K, Solgaard P: Exposure of nickel and the relevance of nickel sensitivity among hospital cleaners. Contact Dermatitis 7:14–18, 1981.
8. Cronin E: Clinical patterns of hand eczema in women. Contact Dermatitis 13:153–161, 1985.
9. Edman B: Sites of contact dermatitis in relationship to particular allergens. Contact Dermatitis 13:129–135, 1985.
10. Edman B, Möller H: Trends and forecasts for standard allergens in a 12-year patch test material. Contact Dermatitis 8:95–104, 1982.
11. Einarsson Ö, Kylin B, Lindstedt G, Wahlberg JE: Chromium, cobalt and nickel in used cutting fluids. Contact Dermatitis 1:182–183, 1975.
12. Emmett EA, Risby TH, Jiang L, et al: Allergic contact dermatitis to nickel: Bioavailability from consumer products and provocation threshold. J Am Acad Dermatol 19:314–322, 1988.
13. Enders F, Przybilla B, Ring J, et al: Epikutantestung mit einer Standardreihe. Hautarzt 39:779–786, 1988.
14. Fischer T: Occupational nickel dermatitis. In Maibach HI, Menné T (eds): Nickel and the Skin: Immunology and Toxicology. Boca Raton, FL, CRC Press, 1989, pp 117–132.
15. Fregert S: Occupational dermatitis in a 10-year material. Contact Dermatitis 1:96–107, 1975.
16. Gammelgaard B, Veien NK: Nickel in nails, hair and plasma from nickel-hypersensitive women. Acta Derm Venereol (Stockh) 70:417–420, 1990.
17. Gawkrodger DJ, Vestey JP, Wong W-K, Buxton PK: Contact clinic survey of nickel-sensitive subjects. Contact Dermatitis 14:165–169, 1986.
18. Goh CL: An epidemiological comparison between occupational and non-occupational hand eczema. Br J Dermatol 120:77–82, 1989.
19. Gola M, Sertoli A, Angelini G, et al: GIRDCA data bank for occupational and environmental contact dermatitis (1984–1988). Am J Contact Dermatitis 3:179–188, 1992.
20. Gollhausen R, Enders F, Przybilla B, et al: Trends in allergic contact sensitization. Contact Dermatitis 18:147–154, 1988.
21. Grandjean P, Nielsen GD, Andersen O: Human nickel exposure and chemobiokinetics. In Maibach HI, Menné T (eds): Nickel and the Skin: Immunology and Toxicology. Boca Raton, FL, CRC Press, 1989, pp 9–34.
22. Handfield-Jones S, Boyle J, Harman RRM: Contact allergy caused by metal sprays. Contact Dermatitis 16:44–45, 1987.
23. Hemingway JD, Molokhia MM: The dissolution of metallic nickel in artificial sweat. Contact Dermatitis 16:99–105, 1987.
24. van Hoogstraten IMW, von Blomberg BME, Boden D, et al: Effects of oral exposure to nickel of chromium on cutaneous sensitization. Curr Probl Dermatol 20:237–241, 1991.

25. Katz SA, Samitz MH: Leaching of nickel from stainless steel consumer commodities. Acta Derm Venereol (Stockh) 55:113–115, 1975.
26. Keczkes K, Basheer AM, Wyatt EH: The persistence of allergic contact sensitivity: A 10-year follow-up in 100 patients. Br J Dermatol 107:461–465, 1982.
27. Lammintausta K, Kalimo K: Nickel sensitivity and the course of atopic dermatitis in adulthood. Contact Dermatitis 22:144–147, 1990.
28. Lammintausta J, Pitkänen O-P, Kalimo K, Jansen CT: Interrelationship of nickel and cobalt contact sensitization. Contact Dermatitis 13:148–152, 1985.
29. Larsson-Stymne B, Widström L: Ear piercing—A cause of nickel allergy in schoolgirls? Contact Dermatitis 13:289–293, 1985.
30. Mastromatteo E: Nickel. Am Ind Hyg Assoc J 47:589–601, 1986.
31. Meding B, Swanbeck G: Occupational hand eczema in an industrial city. Contact Dermatitis 22:13–23, 1990.
32. Menné T: Nickel Allergy [thesis]. University of Copenhagen, Department of Dermatology, Gentofte Hospital, Hellerup, Denmark, 1983.
33. Menné T: Relationship between cobalt and nickel sensitization in females. Contact Dermatitis 6:337–340, 1980.
34. Menné T, Brandrup F, Thestrup-Pedersen K, et al: Patch test reactivity to nickel alloys. Contact Dermatitis 16:255–259, 1987.
35. Menné T, Rasmussen K: Regulation of nickel exposure in Denmark. Contact Dermatitis 23:57–58, 1990.
36. Menné T, Solgaard P: Temperature-dependent nickel release from nickel alloys. Contact Dermatitis 5:82–84, 1979.
37. Menné T, Wilkinson JD: Individual predisposition to contact dermatitis. In Rycroft RJG, Menné T, Frosch PJ, Benezra C (eds): Textbook of Contact Dermatitis. Berlin, Springer-Verlag, 1992, pp 123–130.
38. Möller H, Svensson Å: Metal sensitivity: Positive history but negative test indicates atopy. Contact Dermatitis 14:57–60, 1986.
39. Moorthy TT, Tan GH: Nickel sensitivity in Singapore. Int J Dermatol 25:307–309, 1986.
40. Motolese A, Truzzi M, Giannini A, Seidenari S: Contact dermatitis and contact sensitization among enamellers and decorators in the ceramics industry. Contact Dermatitis 28:59–62, 1993.
41. National Academy of Sciences: Nickel. Washington, DC, National Academy of Sciences, 1975.
42. Nethercott JR, Holness DL: Cutaneous nickel sensitivity in Toronto, Canada. J Am Acad Dermatol 22:756–761, 1990.
43. Nethercott JR, Holness DL, Adams RM, et al: Patch testing with a routine screening tray in North America, 1985 through 1989: II. Gender and response. Am J Contact Dermatitis 2:130–134, 1991.
44. Nethercott JF, Holness DL, Adams RM, et al: Patch testing with a routine screening tray in North America, 1987 through 1989: IV. Occupation and response. Am J Contact Dermatitis 2:247–254, 1991.
45. Niordson A-M: Nickel sensitivity as a cause of rhinitis. Contact Dermatitis 7:273–274, 1981.
46. Pecegueiro M: Contact dermatitis due to nickel in fertilizers. Contact Dermatitis 22:114–115, 1990.
47. Peters K, Gammelgaard B, Menné T: Nickel content of human fingernails as a measure of occupational exposure to nickel. In Frosch PJ, Dooms-Goossens A, Lachapelle J-M, et al (eds): Current Topics in Contact Dermatitis. Berlin, Springer-Verlag, 1989, pp 565–567.
48. Raith L, Jaeger K: The nickel content of chalk—Cause of contact dermatitis? Contact Dermatitis 14:61, 1986.
49. Romaguera C, Grimalt F, Vilaplana J: Contact dermatitis from nickel: An investigation of its sources. Contact Dermatitis 19:52–57, 1988.
50. Rycroft RJG: Occupational contact dermatitis. In Rycroft RJG, Menné T, Frosch PJ, Benezra C (eds): Textbook of Contact Dermatitis. Berlin, Springer-Verlag, 1992, pp 341–399.
51. Rystedt I: Contact sensitivity in adults with atopic dermatitis in childhood. Contact Dermatitis 13:1–8, 1985.
52. Rystedt I, Fischer T: Relationship between nickel and cobalt sensitization in hard metal workers. Contact Dermatitis 9:195–200, 1983.
53. Sunderman FW Jr, Aitio A, Morgan LG, Norseth T: Biological monitoring of nickel. Toxicol Ind Health 2:17–78, 1986.
54. Todd DJ, Burrows D, Stanford CF: Atopy in subjects with a history of nickel allergy but negative patch tests. Contact Dermatitis 21:129–133, 1989.
55. Veien NK, Hattel T, Justesen O, Nørholm A: Why do young girls become nickel sensitive? Contact Dermatitis 15:306–307, 1986.

56. Veien NK, Hattel T, Laurberg G: Patch test results from a private dermatologic practice for two periods of 5 years with a 10-year interval. Am J Contact Dermatitis 3:189–192, 1992.
57. Veien NK, Heydenreich G, Kaaber K, Willumsen P: Hudsygdomme. Arbejdsbetingede hudsygdomme diagnosticeret af hudlæger i Jylland [Occupational skin diseases diagnosed by dermatologists in Jutland]. Copenhagen, Arbejdsmiljøfondet [Industrial Environment Fund], 1986.
58. Wahlberg JE: Nickel: Animal sensitization assays. In Maibach HI, Menné T (eds): Nickel and the Skin: Immunology and Toxicology. Boca Raton, FL, CRC Press, 1989, pp 65–73.
59. Wall LM: Nickel penetration through rubber gloves. Contact Dermatitis 6:461–463, 1980.
60. Wall LM: Spot tests and chemical analyses for allergen evaluation. In Rycroft RJG, Menné T, Frosch PJ, Benezra C (eds): Textbook of Contact Dermatitis. Berlin, Springer-Verlag, 1992, pp 277–285.
61. Wall LM, Calnan CD: Occupational nickel dermatitis in the electroforming industry. Contact Dermatitis 6:414–420, 1980.
62. Wall LM, Gebauer KA: A follow-up study of occupational skin disease in Western Australia. Contact Dermatitis 24:241–243, 1991.
63. Wall LM, Gebauer KA: Occupational skin disease in Western Australia. Contact Dermatitis 24:101–109, 1991.
64. Widström L, Erikssohn I: Nickel allergy and ear piercing in young men. In Frosch PJ, Dooms-Goossens A, Lachapelle J-M, et al (eds): Current Topics in Contact Dermatitis. Berlin, Springer-Verlag, 1989, pp 188–190.
65. Wilkinson DS, Wilkinson JD: Nickel allergy and hand eczema. In Maibach HI, Menné T (eds): Nickel and the Skin: Immunology and Toxicology. Boca Raton, FL, CRC Press, 1989, pp 133–163.
66. World Health Organization. International Agency for Research on Cancer: Chromium, Nickel and Welding. IARC Monographs on the Evaluation of Carcinogenic Risks to Humans, vol 49, 1990.
67. Yang R, Maibach HI: Nickel: Human sensitization assays. In Maibach HI, Menné T (eds): Nickel and the Skin: Immunology and Toxicology. Boca Raton, FL, CRC Press, 1989, pp 75–78.

RIITTA JOLANKI, DTECH (CHEMENG)
LASSE KANERVA, MD, PHD
TUULA ESTLANDER, MD, PHD
KYLLIKKI TARVAINEN, MD

EPOXY DERMATITIS

From the Institute of Occupational Health
Section of Dermatology
Helsinki, Finland

Reprint requests to:
Riitta Jolanki, DTech
Institute of Occupational Health
Section of Dermatology
Topeliuksenkatu 41 a A
FIN-00250
Helsinki, Finland

The most frequent cause of epoxy dermatitis is the use of compounds of the epoxy resin system, which is composed of an epoxy resin and either a hardener, a reactive diluent, a filler, or other additives. Epoxy dermatitis can also be caused by epichlorohydrin and bisphenol A, which are the primary raw materials of epoxy resins; by any other compound containing an epoxy group in its molecule; and by epoxy acrylates.[55]

The first product created that contained epoxy resin was an adhesive, which was introduced in 1946. Large-scale production of epoxy resins began in 1952. Dermatitis caused by exposure to epoxy resin compounds was observed in the 1950s, shortly after epoxy resins were introduced.[17,55]

CHEMISTRY AND PROPERTIES OF EPOXY COMPOUNDS

Epoxy Resin Compounds

EPOXY RESINS

Epoxy resins contain at least two epoxy groups in their molecules. The term "epoxy resin" may refer to the resins in both the uncured thermoplastic and cured thermoset states. The uncured resins can be cross-linked through the use of a variety of curing agents (hardeners) to form cured plastics with insoluble three-dimensional structures. The reaction products of epichlorohydrin and bisphenol A resulted in the first commercial epoxy resins, which are generally mixtures of diglycidyl ether of bisphenol A (DGEBA), with a molecular weight (MW) of 340 and with oligomers with higher MW. The average number of repetitive parts in the oligomers ranges from essentially 0 to approximately 25 (Fig. 1).[6] Resins with a low average MW of 350–400 are liquids with a relatively high viscosity and contain monomeric DGEBA up to more than 90%. Resins with an average MW of more than 900 are solids but may contain even more than 15% DGEBA.[46,55]

DGEBA epoxy resins possess a unique combination of properties, for example, easy cure, low shrinkage, high adhesive strength, high mechanical properties, high electrical insulation, good chemical resistance, and versatility. Special properties of non-DGEBA epoxy resins have made the non-DGEBA epoxy resins competitive with the less expensive DGEBA resins for certain applications. However, the epoxy resin based on DGEBA still forms 75% of the currently used epoxy resins.[78]

Reactive Diluents

Reactive diluents are used to modify epoxy resins, principally by reducing their viscosity. Reactive diluents are generally glycidyl ethers—sometimes glycidyl esters—of aliphatic or aromatic structure, which participate in the cross-linking reactions by their epoxy groups and become chemically linked to cured epoxy resins. Aliphatic diluents include such compounds as *n*-butyl glycidyl ether and 1,4-butanediol diglycidyl ether, whereas phenyl glycidyl ether and cresyl glycidyl ether are good examples of aromatic diluents. More than half of the epoxy resin products studied contained varying amounts of reactive diluents (0.1–20%).[46,58]

Hardeners

When epoxy resins are used in two-component products, the hardeners are added to the resins immediately preceding the application, and the subsequent cross-linking occurs at either an ambient or an elevated temperature. One-component products contain latent curing agents, which are inactive at normal storage temperatures but which initiate the cross-linking when heated. Examples of one-component products are epoxy or epoxy-polyester powder paints[82] and one-pack glues.[20]

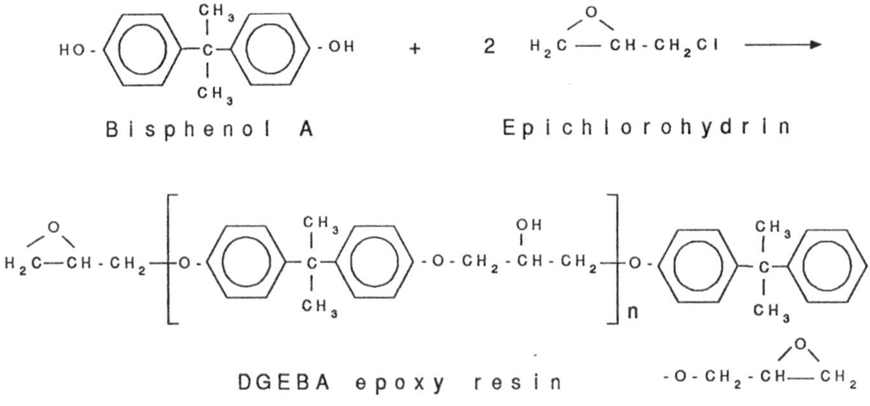

FIGURE 1. DGEBA epoxy resin.

Currently, a wide variety of curing agents are available. Aliphatic amines include, for example, ethylene diamine, diethylene triamine, and triethylene tetramine; isophorone diamine is a cycloaliphatic amine, and 4,4′-diaminodiphenyl methane belongs to the group of aromatic amines.[78] Aliphatic and cycloaliphatic amines are low-viscosity liquids that react readily with epoxy resins at ambient temperatures; less reactive aromatic amines require an elevated curing temperature.[78]

Polyamines are often troublesome to work with because of their reactivity and volatility and also because of their irritating and sensitizing properties to the skin and respiratory tract. To overcome these problems, less volatile and less reactive polyamides and amine-epoxy adducts have been developed. Polyamides are prepared by combining aliphatic amines (e.g., diethylene triamine or triethylene tetramine) with fatty acids. Amine-epoxy adducts are formed in a reaction between epoxy resin and an excess of polyamine, mostly diethylene triamine, triethylene tetramine, or isophorone diamine.[6] In the amine-epoxy adduct hardeners used in metal paints, the content of free amine is about 5%, but for those used in floor and concrete coatings, the corresponding value is about 20%. Free DGEBA is not found in amine-epoxy adducts.[46,55] When DGEBA epoxy resins are cured by polyamine-bearing hardeners at room temperature, the amounts of unreacted DGEBA and polyamine diminish rapidly within one to two days, but thereafter the decrease is slow. Nevertheless, after one week's cure, 0.02–12% of free DGEBA and 0.01–1% of free diethylene triamine were found when six different epoxy resin products were experimentally cured by diethylene triamine.[45]

Tertiary polyamines, for example, 2,4,6-tris-(dimethylaminomethyl)phenol (tris-DMP), are catalyst-type curing agents used for epoxy resin homopolymerization.[78] In six epoxy paint hardeners analyzed, the content of tris-DMP was 0–9%.[64] Organic anhydride hardeners are used when good electrical properties are required. With the anhydrides the cross-linking reaction is catalyzed by tertiary amines, and an elevated curing temperature (50–200°C) is used. The anhydrides include, for example, phthalic anhydride and phthalic anhydride derivatives.[55,78] Typical latent curing agents in powder paints are composed of about 4% hardeners, such as dicyandiamide or pyromellitic anhydride. The polymerization is achieved in a curing oven at about 200°C.[82]

Epoxy Acrylates

The first epoxy acrylate, known as BIS-GMA (2,2-bis[4-(2-hydroxy-3-methacryloxy-propoxy)phenyl]propane) was developed by Bowen in 1956 when he incorporated glycidyl methacrylate containing an epoxy group into bisphenol A. Dental composite resin products based on BIS-GMA have been used in dental restoration work since 1962.[101] BIS-GMA or other epoxy acrylates, also called vinyl esters, can also be manufactured by combining DGEBA or other epoxy resins and methacrylic acid or other (meth)acrylic acids, respectively.[3,6] Epoxy acrylates have the desirable properties of both epoxy resins and polyacrylates, for example, a relatively low volumetric shrinkage during the curing process, as in epoxy resins, and an adequate polymerization rate, as in methacrylates of low molecular mass.[54,101]

The polymerization of epoxy acrylates is activated either chemically by peroxides and tertiary amines or by visible or ultraviolet light. Chemically cured dental restorative composite material is available in two BIS-GMA-based components. The tooth-colored base paste contains a tertiary amine (1–2%), and the catalyst paste contains dibenzoyl peroxide (1–1.5%). The light-cured composite material consists of only one BIS-GMA-based component. In the manufacture of reinforced plastic products, the vinyl ester resins are used after being dissolved in styrene.[3,54]

Other Epoxy Compounds

Apart from epoxy resins, epoxy reactive diluents, and epichlorohydrin, other compounds containing at least one epoxy group in their molecules are reactive substances and are able to react with proteins, but the compounds are not otherwise chemically closely related. Dermatologically interesting examples of the compounds are triglycidyl isocyanurate (TGIC),[81] 2,3-epoxypropyl trimethyl ammonium chloride,[27] and *trans*-methyl-3-(4-methoxyphenyl)glycidate.[15]

USE OF EPOXY COMPOUNDS

Epoxy Resin Compounds

Of the total world production of epoxy resins—more than 500,000 tons a year—about 45% are used in coatings, and the remainder (55%) in structural applications.[6,55,78] The scope of epoxy resin application is broad. Epoxy resins are used to provide good resistance against heat, water, and most chemicals and to form tough, high-strength adhesive bonds on metal and other surfaces (e.g., plastics, rubber, wood, glass, and ceramics). They are used to insulate and encapsulate, as well as in the assembly of a wide variety of electrical and electronic devices and in the manufacture of plastic items, such as sporting goods. They are also used in reinforced plastics or composites and in casting, molding, and tooling.[6,55,78,94]

Most epoxy surface coatings are based on DGEBA epoxy resins. Liquid epoxy resins are used in two-component solventless coatings. Waterborne epoxy coatings are prepared by the dispersion of epoxy resins modified with water-soluble functional groups or by the emulsification of DGEBA epoxy resins with surfactants.[78] Both solventless and solvent-borne epoxy coatings have been employed mainly as anticorrosion protection for metals (e.g., marine and maintenance coatings), as waterproof protection for concrete, and as chemical-resistant protection for floors and walls.[6,78] Two-component coatings can be cured at ambient temperatures with polyamines, polyamides, and amine-epoxy adducts. Tertiary amines (e.g., tris-DMP) are frequently used to accelerate the curing rates.[64] Powder epoxy paints include solid DGEBA epoxy resins mixed with a curing agent and an accelerator.[82]

Epoxy adhesives are widely used as two-component, ambient-cure, general adhesives in domestic applications—as in two-tube epoxy kits—and also in industrial applications. Liquid DGEBA epoxy resins are used to formulate most of the one- and two-component epoxy adhesives. The curing agent generally consists of polyamides or aliphatic polyamines (e.g., diethylene triamine and triethylene tetramine). Epoxy adhesives can be formulated with reactive diluents to give mixtures a low viscosity with improved wetting, spreading, and penetrating action.[89]

Reinforced plastics are combinations of strong, continuous glass and carbon fibers and polymeric binders. Glass fibers, woven cloth, and roving and chopped mat can be impregnated with an epoxy resin/curing agent matrix. Epoxy composites made with glass fibers usually have a DGEBA epoxy resin/diamine matrix. Epoxy composites are used in sporting goods such as tennis racket frames, ski poles, and fishing rods; in the automotive, boatbuilding, and aircraft industries; and in military and aerospace applications.[16,68,78,94] Epoxy resins can also be used as sizing agents for the continuous glass fibers used in polyester composites.[59]

Casting resins are liquid and solventless mixtures of low-molecular-mass epoxy resin, a curing agent, and additives (e.g., fillers, reinforcements, and catalysts). The mixture is poured into molds and cured to solid structures. The casting resins are used mainly as electrical insulating material in the manufacture of transformers, switching gear, circuit breakers, conductors, and insulators. Anhydride-cured cycloaliphatic epoxy resins are commonly used to improve arc-track resistance and weatherability (e.g., in outdoor electrical insulators).[62,78]

Epoxy molding compounds are solid mixtures of epoxy resin (e.g., epoxy novolac), a curing agent and catalyst, mold-release compounds, fillers, and other additives. The molding compounds become liquid at relatively low temperatures (150–200° C). Epoxy molding compounds are used, for example, in the manufacture of models and engine covers and in the encapsulation of electrical components.[1,55,78]

Epoxy resins were introduced in 1956 in the preparation of samples for electron microscopy, and they are still widely used today.[39,56] Three types of epoxy resin are used: the DGEBA epoxy resins, the diglycidyl and triglycidyl ethers of diols and polyols, and low-viscosity resin of vinyl cyclohexane dioxide. The epoxy resins are generally hardened by anhydrides (e.g., dodecenyl succinic anhydride), using amines (e.g., tris-DMP) as accelerators.[22,39,56]

Epoxy Acrylates

BIS-GMA is used in dental fillings and coating materials, in dentin primers,[63] and in sealing the fissures in posterior teeth in order to protect those teeth from caries.[54] Epoxy acrylates also have many industrial applications. They are used in ultraviolet curable printing inks and coatings[10,24]; in corrosion-resistant equipment, body, and structural parts for land transportation equipment; in electrical insulation for heavy electrical equipment; and in marine applications.[3,94]

Other Epoxy Compounds

TGIC is used mainly in thermosetting one-component polyester powder coatings as a hardener[78] but is also used in electrical insulation materials, resin molding systems, laminated sheetings, printing circuits, tools, inks, adhesives, lining materials, stabilizers for plastics, and amine captures.[81] Two,3-epoxypropyl trimethyl ammonium chloride is used in the manufacture of cationic starch as a cationizing chemical and in the manufacture of ion-exchange resins.[8,27] Epoxy compounds are also used in drug syntheses.[15,87] They can also be found among the oxidation products of abietic and related acids.[44]

DELAYED ALLERGIC EPOXY DERMATITIS

Epoxy Resin Compounds

The first reports of sensitization to epoxy compounds were published in the 1950s in Switzerland, the Netherlands, the United States, and Great Britain, where most of the epoxy resin development had taken place.[17,55]

Diglycidyl Ether of Bisphenol A (DGEBA) Epoxy Resins

The highly alkaline amine hardeners were first considered to be responsible for most cases of dermatitis and sensitization observed during the handling of components of the epoxy system,[9,12] but later, Thorgeirsson and Fregert confirmed that the main sensitizer was DGEBA (i.e., DGEBA-based epoxy resin oligomer with an MW of 340).[97] In the guinea pig maximization test, the oligomer with an MW of 624 was also a sensitizer, but it had minor sensitizing capacity, whereas oligomers with an MW of more than 900 did not produce sensitivity.[98]

Up to 1964, 1.6% of 1,690 patients who were not employed in the epoxy resin industry developed allergic patch test reactions to DGEBA epoxy resin at the Department of Dermatology of the University of Lund.[35] Thus the DGEBA epoxy resin, because it is one of the top 20 contact allergens, was included in the European standard patch test series in 1966.[55] In the 1970s and 1980s, the North American Contact Dermatitis Group studied about 9,000 patients and found that 2–3% were allergic to the standard epoxy resin.[71,86,92] Edman found a lower frequency—of 1%—among 3,562 patients patch tested during 1982–1987 at the Malmö General Hospital in Sweden.[23] A frequency of 3.7% was found among patients in Finland and in Canada, corresponding to the selectivity of patients in occupational dermatology clinics.[52,55]

Wilkinson et al. detected contact allergy to epoxy resin in 2.9% of their tested patients with occupational skin diseases,[103] and Fregert found epoxy resin allergy in 5.1% of his male patients with occupational dermatoses.[32] The proportion of cases induced by epoxy resin compounds was 7.2% at the Institute of Occupational Health in Helsinki.[55] After chromium and rubber chemicals, epoxy resin compounds are the third most frequent cause of occupational allergic dermatoses[26,61]; they have induced occupational allergic contact dermatitis in 11.7–12.5% of patients.[52,55]

Allergic contact dermatitis caused by epoxy resin is often due to exposure to two-component glues and bonding agents.[1,31,55] One patient, a floor layer, became sensitized from a one-pack epoxy glue.[20] Even small amounts in ready products are sufficient to cause sensitization, for example, contaminants in hand-applied eye lenses[43] and clothing.[74] There are also several reports of workers sensitized to epoxy resins used as binders in carbon or glass fiber reinforced plastics products.[13,16,18,21,51,76,93] Epoxy resin used as a sizing agent in glass fibers may induce contact allergy.[59] Epoxy resins used in electron microscopy have caused a few cases of allergic sensitization.[22] Contact sensitivity from epoxy resin in medical equipment has been reported.[2,,11,38,75,85,99] Allergic contact dermatitis has also been induced by unhardened epoxy resin in some other finished products.[1,28,34,48,73] Epoxy resins used as stabilizers and plasticizers for polyvinyl chloride have been shown to be sensitizers.[1,2,99] In addition, a few cases of allergic contact dermatitis due to DGEBA epoxy resins with a high average MW have been reported,[20,58,93] even though the amount of DGEBA has been as low as 0.2% in the causative products.[58]

Non-diglycidyl Ether of Bisphenol A (non-DGEBA) Epoxy Resins

Most of those who have contact allergy to epoxy resins have been sensitized to DGEBA epoxy resins.[1,31,55] Since the 1980s, allergic contact dermatitis has also been reported from non-DGEBA epoxy resins such as N-N′-tetraglycidyl-4,4′-methylene dianiline and *ortho*-diglycidyl phthalate,[4,16] 4-glycidyloxy-N,N-diglycidylaniline,[76] vinyl cyclohexane dioxide,[22] and a triglycidyl derivative of *para*-aminophenol.[4] In addition, cycloaliphatic epoxy resins based on diglycidyl ester of hexahydrophthalic acid, heterocyclic dimethyl hydantoin epoxy resins, phenol novolac epoxy resins, and brominated epoxy resins have been found to be causes of allergic contact dermatitis.[57,58,62] Many of the patients sensitized to non-DGEBA epoxy resins do not have contact allergy to DGEBA epoxy resin.

Reactive Diluents

An investigation by Fregert and Rorsman emphasized the occurrence of contact allergy to reactive diluents in patients allergic to epoxy resins.[35] Epoxy reactive diluents have been revealed to be strong sensitizers in guinea pigs and in humans.[55,57,61,79,95] Reactive diluents are as common contact allergens as hardeners among patients exposed to an epoxy resin system,[55,100] and contact allergy to reactive diluents without contact allergy to epoxy resins is possible.[57,61,79] Most patients sensitized to reactive diluents are allergic to phenyl glycidyl ether, cresyl glycidyl ether, hexanediol diglycidyl ether, butanediol diglycidyl ether, or butyl glycidyl ether, and cross-sensitization between reactive diluents is common.[55,57,100]

Hardeners

In several investigations since the 1950s, polyamine hardeners have been found to be contact irritants and sensitizers.[12,17] In the guinea pig maximization test, polyamine hardeners with a low MW were found to be strong sensitizers.[96] Most of the patients with contact allergy to epoxy hardeners react to 4,4′-diaminodiphenyl methane, diethylene triamine, and triethylene tetramine.[55,100] In addition, cases of contact allergy to isophorone diamine,[1,31,42,64] trimethyl hexamethylene diamine,[64] or xylylene diamine[64,84] have been reported. Polyamides and amine-epoxy adducts induced sensitization probably only due to the polyamine remnants.[64,96] Isolated contact allergy to epoxy hardeners is unusual, but possible.[64,100] Tris-DMP has been reported to be probably a more common allergen than expected.[64] Sporadic reports of contact allergy to nonamine hardeners have been published in the case of a latent curing agent—dicyandiamide[90]—and an anhydride hardener—dodecenyl succinic anhydride.[40]

Allergic patch test reactions to 4,4′-diaminodiphenyl methane or ethylene diamine are not necessarily an indication of sensitivity from exposure to epoxy resin hardeners. The relevancy of 4,4′-diaminodiphenyl methane allergy is sometimes difficult to detect. For example, a positive patch test reaction to 4,4′-diaminodiphenyl methane may represent allergy to *para*-amino compounds (e.g., *para*-phenylene diamine)[36] or exposure to diphenyl methane diisocyanate.[61] Ethylene diamine allergy may be due to exposure, for example, to rubber, synthetic coolants, or topical creams.[29]

Epichlorohydrin and Bisphenol A

Occupational contact dermatitis due to epichlorohydrin and bisphenol A is uncommon.[55] In the finished DGEBA epoxy resin, the proportion of free epichlorohydrin is less than 0.001%. The proportion of bisphenol A is even smaller, because in the manufacturing process, epichlorohydrin is always present in excess to ensure that the molecules terminate in epoxy groups. In epoxy resin plants, despite closed manufacturing systems, workers may get sensitized to epichlorohydrin, but they do not generally become sensitized to bisphenol A.[102] Allergy to epichlorohydrin has also been reported from a solvent cement[7] and from drug synthesis of propranolol hydrochloride and oxprenolol hydrochloride.[83] Epichlorohydrin at 1% in petrolatum can also induce active sensitization in patch testing.[55]

Cases of allergy to bisphenol A have been reported, for example from semisynthetic waxes,[30] plastic footwear,[91] and BIS-GMA-based dental composite resins containing 0.014–0.015% bisphenol A.[55] In some studies, a high incidence of bisphenol A allergy was found among those sensitized to epoxy resin.[37,69] These results have not, however, been confirmed by other investigations.[55,102] The contact allergy to bisphenol A may also be a cross-reaction with compounds responsible for phenol formaldehyde resin allergy, such as dihydroxydiphenyl methanes (bisphenol F).[14,61]

Epoxy Acrylates

The guinea pig maximization test has shown that epoxy acrylates are weak to extreme sensitizers.[10] Despite the increasing use of epoxy acrylates in dental care and in industry, relatively few reports on contact allergy due to these compounds have been published.[10,24,63,80] The sensitized subjects have mainly been workers in the ultraviolet-light printing industry[10,24,80] or in dental nursing.[63] Work in the manufacture of ultraviolet-curable epoxy acrylate paints can also induce contact allergy.[55] Patients who acquire their epoxy acrylate allergy from dental composite resins that contain BIS-GMA as the main monomer are in general concomitantly allergic to both BIS-GMA and the standard epoxy resin.[63] Contact allergy to epoxy acrylates has also been found in patients who had been exposed to DGEBA epoxy resins but who had no known exposure to the epoxy acrylates.[61,64,66]

Other Epoxy Compounds

TGIC is a known skin irritant[81] but has recently been shown to be an allergen as well.[60,81] Workers may become sensitized to TGIC from short-term exposure to the chemical in the production of TGIC, in the manufacture and use of TGIC-containing polyester powder paints, and in the manufacture of circuit boards[60,77,81] (Figs. 2 and 3). Two,3-epoxypropyl trimethyl ammonium chloride has been shown

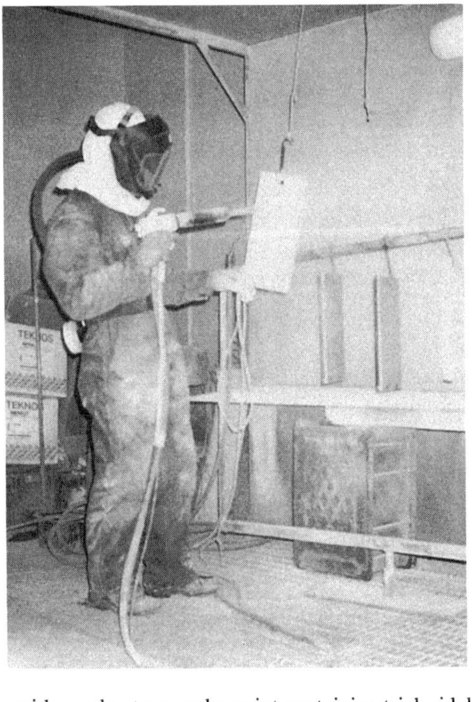

FIGURE 2. Painting with a polyester powder paint containing triglycidyl isocyanurate (TGIC).

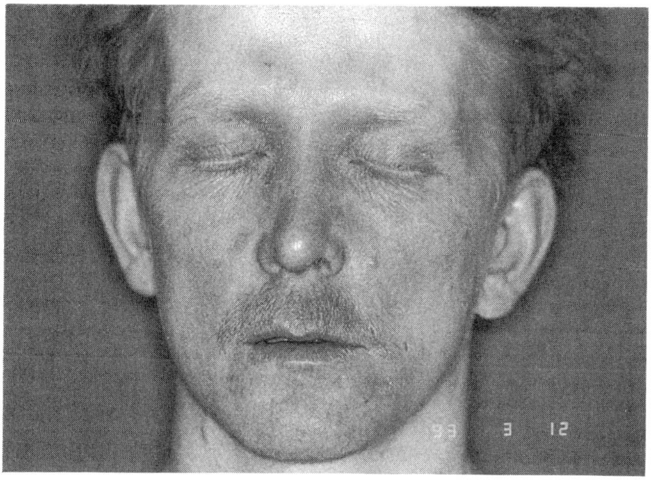

FIGURE 3. Face dermatitis caused by contact allergy to triglycidyl isocyanurate (TGIC) in powder paints.

to be a moderate sensitizer in guinea pigs and to cause allergic contact dermatitis in humans.[8,27] In all cases, sensitization took place after a short period of contact with the chemical. An intermediate product in the synthesis of the drug diltiazem hydrochloride, 2,3-epoxy-3-(4-methoxyphenyl)propionate has induced contact allergy in two cases.[15,87] Another epoxy compound, 13,14-epoxyabietic acid, is a sensitizer in guinea pigs.[44]

IMMEDIATE ALLERGIC EPOXY DERMATITIS

Contact urticaria can be caused by aliphatic polyamine hardeners.[29] In a 1974 report, a patch test with an epoxy resin induced generalized urticaria.[104] In 1983, Suhonen reported on two patients who showed in a patch test immediate urticarial reactions to a DGEBA epoxy resin used in a ski pole factory, but the DGEBA epoxy resin in the patch test standard series did not give an immediate reaction. The causative agent was not further identified. In addition to contact urticaria, another immediate-type allergic disorder induced by epoxy resins is bronchial asthma, which was verified for two patients, who had allergic contact dermatitis due to the resins, too.[66] Prick tests and specific immunoglobulin E determinations indicated that the DGEBA was the specific immediate-type allergen in the two asthma patients. Only two cases of allergic-type dermatoses (i.e., contact urticaria) due to organic phthalic anhydride hardeners have been reported,[58,61] though the anhydrides are well-known occupational respiratory allergens.[67]

IRRITANT EPOXY DERMATITIS

Irritative low-molecular-degradation products may be produced in the tooling of epoxy products and in heating processes.[25] Amine and anhydride hardeners and epichlorohydrin irritate the skin and conjunctivas. In addition to causing irritant contact dermatitis, epichlorohydrin, as a highly reactive compound, and aliphatic polyamines, as highly alkaline compounds (pH 13–14), can cause corrosive burns on the skin.[1,53] Ippen and Mathies described protracted chemical burns minutes or several hours after the exposure of five patients to epichlorohydrin.[53]

DGEBA epoxy resins are not strong irritants, and the irritability decreases with an increasing MW of the oligomer.[49] Curing agents in powder paints, such as dicyandiamide and organic anhydrides, are potentially irritant.[67,82] For four patients, irritant contact dermatitis was caused by DGEBA epoxy resins with a high average MW in paints or paint raw materials; for one patient it was due to a mixture of a DGEBA epoxy resin with a low average MW and its anhydride hardener, used in electrical insulation.[58,61]

OTHER EPOXY DERMATITIS

Purpuric allergic contact dermatitis, sclerodermalike disorders, atypical psoriasis, and erythema multiforme have been described from epoxy compounds.[52] Bachurzewska and Borucka reported Raynaud's-disease-type ailments.[5] Rycroft reported on a patient whose epoxy resin sensitization was followed by atypical psoriasis,[88] and Lichter et al. on a patient whose epoxy resin and hardener was followed by lichenoid contact dermatitis.[70] Photosensitivity has been reported in relation to the heating of DGEBA epoxy resin and the use of epoxy powder paints.[41] Photosensitivity is considered to be probably due to bisphenol A contained in the resin.[72]

INVESTIGATION OF EPOXY DERMATITIS

Exposure

In Finland, 1% of the exposed workers developed an occupational dermatosis due to epoxy resin compounds. Even higher risks of dermatitis from exposure to epoxy resin compounds are found among individual groups of workers constantly exposed to epoxy resin compounds.[57,62] The epoxy resin compounds were revealed to be the main cause for the current dermatosis in 41% of the cases investigated for suspected occupational skin disease and who had a current or previous occupational exposure to epoxy resin compounds.[61]

Epoxy resin compounds have been found to be allergens, especially in painting and paint processing, electrical insulation, gluing, and the manufacture of epoxy objects. In addition to the amount of epoxy resin compounds used, other important aspects in the development of dermatitis from epoxy resin compounds include frequency of skin contacts with the causative agent, concentration of the epoxy compound used, size of the contaminated skin area, and possibilities to use protective gloves.[55] Most of the patients contracting an epoxy compound dermatosis are men.[32,55,71,103] The difference in the frequency of dermatosis between the two genders probably represents differences in exposure.

The identification of specific allergens is especially important in occupational dermatology. First, significant economic issues are connected with occupational disease legislation. Second, prevention of occupational allergic contact dermatitis is possible only when the actual allergen has been identified. It is necessary to combine chemical and dermatological experiences for the optimal investigation of occupational skin diseases induced by epoxy compounds. The methods include patch testing, clarification of the causative agents, and planning of preventive measures for both the patient and, especially, the still healthy fellow workers. In problematic cases, consultations with industrial hygienists, visits to patients' work sites, and analyses of the materials handled by patients are important.[55] Thin-layer chromatography and other chromatographic methods (gas chromatography and high-performance liquid chromatography) can be used to demonstrate the presence or absence of particular allergens.[4,33,56,64]

Location of Dermatitis

Epoxy compounds can induce either direct or airborne contact dermatitis, but the skin symptoms are located mainly on patients' hands or arms. The fingers and interdigital spaces, on the hands; the forearms and wrists, on the arms; and the eyelids, on the face, are the most typical localizations of the skin disorders due to epoxy compounds.[61] Reactive diluents and hardeners have been considered the most probable causes of airborne epoxy resin compound dermatitis because those substances are more volatile than DGEBA epoxy resins.[19] In another study, facial dermatitis was found in 60% of the patients, but it was not especially common among patients allergic to reactive diluents or hardeners.[61]

Skin Testing

No single chemical can be used alone to screen for sensitization to several different contact allergens of epoxy compounds. For instance, of the patients who have developed contact allergy to epoxy resin compounds, 30% are found to be sensitive to more than one of the three main epoxy resin compound groups (i.e., resins, hardeners, and reactive diluents).[55,100] In addition, individual contact allergies to hardeners, reactive diluents, and non-DGEBA epoxy resins are common among workers exposed to epoxy resin compounds.[55] Thus it is highly recommended that patients suspected of contracting contact dermatitis from epoxy resin compounds be tested not only with the standard epoxy resin but also with the individual allergenic compounds, hardeners, reactive diluents, and non-DGEBA epoxy resins according to the contents of the epoxy resin compounds used by those patients. Despite the use of an extensive epoxy compound patch test series, testing with all materials to which patients have been exposed is important, but it should be borne in mind that testing only with the patients' own materials is not always completely reliable, because the allergens may become too diluted and thus give negative patch test results.[55]

A patch test concentration of 0.5% in petrolatum for non-DGEBA epoxy resins is probably preferable to 1% when low-viscosity resins are being tested, because 1% non-DGEBA may irritate.[62] Patch testing with the resinous part alone does not exclude contact allergy to reactive diluents if the patient is also sensitive to the resin. A test concentration of 0.25% in petrolatum was found suitable for testing reactive diluents.[55]

On patch testing, cross allergy has been found between compounds that are closely related chemically, especially between reactive diluents. In addition, patients who are allergic to cycloaliphatic epoxy resins often react to reactive diluents, and vice versa.[55] Patients who react to reactive diluents in the patch testing do not always react to the standard epoxy resin based on DGEBA, even though they have been exposed to the DGEBA epoxy resin. Thus reactive diluents do not produce cross allergy with DGEBA epoxy resins, and contact allergy to reactive diluents is not revealed by testing with the standard epoxy resin. However, an allergic patch test reaction to reactive diluents may also indicate allergy to cycloaliphatic epoxy resins because of cross allergy.[62]

Three reactive diluents (*n*-butyl glycidyl ether, *ortho*-cresyl glycidyl ether, and phenyl glycidyl ether) are available from the test substance suppliers. Aromatic compounds, especially phenyl glycidyl ether, have been found to give an allergic patch test reaction in most of the patients who were allergic to reactive diluents. Of the aliphatic compounds, 1,4-butanediol diglycidyl ether was found to screen contact allergy to reactive diluents better than *n*-butyl glycidyl ether. Thus phenyl glycidyl ether and 1,4-butanediol diglycidyl ether are recommended for patch testing to detect contact allergy due to reactive diluents. Because of common cross-reactivity, the two reactive diluents are probably enough to screen for contact allergy to other related compounds also.[55]

Patch testing with diethylene triamine, triethylene tetramine, 4,4′-diamino-diphenyl methane, isophorone diamine, and tris-DMP should be performed when allergy to epoxy hardeners is suspected. All but tris-DMP are available from the test substance suppliers. The recommended test concentration for tris-DMP is 1% in petrolatum.[64] Because of the vast variety of hardeners used, it is highly recommended to test patients also with the hardeners they have been exposed to; then, test concentrations of up to 10% should be used for the amine-epoxy adducts. A test concentration of about 1% is the most suitable for polyamine-type hardeners.[55]

BIS-GMA and 2,2-bis(4-[2-hydroxy-3-acryloxypropoxy]phenyl)propane (BIS-GA) can be recommended for the detection of contact allergy due to epoxy acrylates. An allergic reaction produced by the standard epoxy resin may indicate contact allergy to epoxy acrylates, and this possibility should be clarified by additional patch tests.[55,63]

In general, petrolatum seems to be a good vehicle for epoxy resin compounds. For solid materials containing uncured epoxy resins, it is preferable to use acetone instead of water so as to soften the material in the patch test chamber.[61]

TREATMENT AND PREVENTION OF EPOXY DERMATITIS

Complete avoidance of contact with the causative allergens is always necessary. In a patient highly sensitive to epoxy compounds, even a minimal amount of allergen may be enough to evoke symptoms on the exposed skin. Most patients who have acquired occupational epoxy dermatitis have to quit their work. Quitting may also be beneficial for prevention of possible respiratory allergy followed by skin sensitization.[66] Allergic epoxy dermatitis nevertheless has a good prognosis. It is easier to avoid contact with less commonly used allergens such as uncured or reactive epoxy compounds than it is to avoid contact with a widespread allergen such as nickel. Skin problems caused by contact with epoxy compounds generally clear up shortly after exposure has ended.[27,50,62]

Those working with epoxy compounds should be aware of the risk of sensitization. Gloves of laminated, multilayered plastic (4H-glove), containing ethylene-vinyl alcohol copolymer, developed especially for the handling of epoxy compounds, give the best protection against them.[47] The use of any type of glove, however, seems to reduce exposure to epoxy resin compounds and helps to protect against the risk of sensitization, although the use of protective gloves may in some individual cases even promote contact allergens to come into contact with the skin.[61] Unhealthy skin, including even small wounds and abrasions, should be protected from epoxy compound exposure because of increased skin penetration. The airways should also be protected from exposure to epoxy compounds, because such compounds can be considered potential causes of asthma. An automatic process as such does not guarantee protection against skin contact and exposure of the respiratory tract with the compounds because of exposure, for example, during maintenance, repair, or sampling.[55]

REFERENCES

1. Adams RM: Occupational Skin Disease. New York, Grune & Stratton, 1983, pp 238–266.

2. Ancona A, Arévalo A, Macotela E: Contact dermatitis in hospital patients. Dermatol Clin 8:95–105, 1990.
3. Anderson TF, Messick VB: Vinyl ester resins. In Pritchard G (ed): Developments in reinforced plastics, Vol 1. London, Elsevier Applied Science Publishers, 1985, pp 29–58.
4. Ayala F, Lembo G, Balato N, et al: The use of laboratory methods in contact dermatitis induced by composite materials. Contact Dermatitis 22:262–266, 1990 [erratum: Contact Dermatitis 23:384, 1990].
5. Bachurzewska B, Borucka I: Gefässläsionen bei Eisenbahnarbeiterinnen, die mit Epoxidharzen in Berührung kommen. Dermatosen 34:77–79, 1986.
6. Bauer RS: Epoxy resins. In Tess RW, Poehlein GW (eds): Applied Polymer Science, 2nd ed. Washington, DC, American Chemical Society, 1985, pp 931–961.
7. Beck MH, King CM: Allergic contact dermatitis to epichlorhydrin in a solvent cement. Contact Dermatitis 9:315, 1983.
8. Bergquist-Karlsson A: Contact allergy to glycidyl trimethyl ammonium chloride. Contact Dermatitis 12:61–62, 1985.
9. Birmingham DJ: Clinical observations on the cutaneous effects associated with curing epoxy resins. Arch Ind Health 19:365–367, 1959.
10. Björkner B: Sensitizing capacity of ultraviolet curable acrylic compounds [doctoral dissertation]. Lund, Sweden, University of Lund, 1984.
11. Boom BW, van Driel LMJ: Allergic contact dermatitis to epoxy resin in infusion sets of an insulin pump. Contact Dermatitis 12:280, 1985.
12. Bourne LB, Milner FJM, Alberman KB: Health problems of epoxy resins and amine-curing agents. Br J Ind Med 16:81–97, 1959.
13. Bruze M, Almgren G: Occupational dermatoses in workers exposed to epoxy-impregnated fiberglass fabric. Dermatosen 37:171–176, 1989.
14. Bruze M, Zimerson E: Contact allergy to dihydroxydiphenyl methanes (bisphenol F). Dermatosen 33:216–220, 1985.
15. Buisson H, Vaillant L, Lasfargues G, et al: Occupational contact dermatitis from *trans*-methyl-3(4-methoxyphenyl)glycidate. Contact Dermatitis 25:262–263, 1991.
16. Burrows D, Fregert S, Campbell H, Trulsson L: Contact dermatitis from the epoxy resins tetraglycidyl-4,4′-methylene dianiline and *o*-diglycidyl phthalate in composite material. Contact Dermatitis 11:80–82, 1984.
17. Calnan CD: Studies in contact dermatitis. Trans St Johns Hosp Dermatol Soc 40:12–19, 1958.
18. Conde-Salazar L, Guimaraens D, Romero LV, et al: Occupational dermatitis from glass fiber. Contact Dermatitis 13:195–196, 1985.
19. Dahlquist I, Fregert S: Allergic contact dermatitis from volatile epoxy hardeners and reactive diluents. Contact Dermatitis 5:406–407, 1979.
20. Dahlquist I, Fregert S, Persson K, Trulsson L: Epoxy resin in a one-pack glue. Contact Dermatitis 5:189–190, 1979.
21. Dahlquist I, Fregert S, Trulsson L: Allergic contact dermatitis from epoxy resin finished glass fiber. Contact Dermatitis 5:190, 1979.
22. Dannaker CJ: Allergic sensitization to a non-bisphenol A epoxy of the cycloaliphatic class. J Occup Med 30:641–643, 1988.
23. Edman B: Computerized patch data in contact allergy [doctoral dissertation]. Malmö, Sweden, Lund University, 1988.
24. Emmett EA, Kominsky JR: Allergic contact dermatitis from ultraviolet cured ink. J Occup Med 19:113–115, 1977.
25. Engström B, Henriks-Eckerman M-L: Hitsaustyö ja maali [Welding and paint]. Helsinki, Työterveyslaitos, Työolot 68, 1988.
26. Estlander T: Occupational skin disease in Finland: Observations made during 1974–88 at the Institute of Occupational Health, Helsinki. Acta Derm Venerol 155(Suppl):1–85,1990.
27. Estlander T, Jolanki R, Kanerva L: Occupational dermatitis to 2,3-epoxypropyl trimethyl ammonium chloride. Contact Dermatitis 14:49–52, 1986.
28. Fischer T, Fregert S, Thulin I, Trulsson L: Unhardened epoxy resin in tool handles. Contact Dermatitis 16:45, 1987.
29. Fisher AA: Contact Dermatitis, 3rd ed. Philadelphia, Lea & Febiger, 1986.
30. Freeman K, Warin AP: Contact dermatitis due to bisphenol A in semi-synthetic waxes. Contact Dermatitis 11:259–260, 1984.
31. Fregert S: Contact dermatitis from epoxy resin systems. In Maibach HI (ed): Occupational and Industrial Dermatology, 2nd ed. Chicago, Year Book, 1987, pp 341–345.
32. Fregert S: Occupational dermatitis in a 10-year material. Contact Dermatitis 1:96–107, 1975.

33. Fregert S: Physicochemical methods for detection of contact allergens. Dermatol Clin 6:97–104, 1988.
34. Fregert S, Orsmark K: Allergic contact dermatitis due to epoxy resin in textile labels. Contact Dermatitis 11:131–132, 1984.
35. Fregert S, Rorsman H: Allergens in epoxy resins. Acta Allergol 19:296–299, 1964.
36. Gailhofer G, Ludvan M: Zur Wertigkeit positiver Epikutantestreaktionen auf 4,4′-Diaminodiphenylmethan. Dermatosen 37:17–22, 1989.
37. Gaul LE: Sensitivity to bisphenol A. Arch Dermatol 82:1003, 1960.
38. Geldof BA, Oranje AP, van Joost T: Hand eczema associated with continuous subcutaneous insulin infusion. Contact Dermatitis 20:384–385, 1989.
39. Glauert AM: Epoxy resins: An update on their selection and use. Eur Microscopy Anal Sept:13–18, 1991.
40. Göransson K: Allergic contact dermatitis to an epoxy hardener: Dodecenyl-succinic anhydride. Contact Dermatitis 3:277–278, 1977.
41. Göransson K, Andersson R, Andersson G, et al: An outbreak of occupational photodermatosis of the face in a factory in northern Sweden. In Berglund B, Lindvall T, Sundell J (eds): Indoor Air, Vol 3. Stockholm, Swedish Council for Building Research, 1984, pp 367–375.
42. Guerra L, Vincenzi C, Bardazzi F, Tosti A: Contact sensitization due to isophoronediamine. Contact Dermatitis 27:52–53, 1992.
43. Hambly EM, Wilkinson DS: Unusual presentation of epoxy resin sensitivity. Contact Dermatitis 4:114, 1978.
44. Hausen BM, Krohn K, Budianto E: Contact allergy due to colophony: VII. Sensitizing studies with oxidation products of abietic and related acids. Contact Dermatitis 23:352–358, 1990.
45. Henriks-Eckerman M-L, Laijoki T: Alifaattisten polyamiinien ja epoksioligomeerien sitoutuminen kylmäkovettumisessa [Aliphatic polyamines and epoxy oligomers in cold cured epoxy products]. Työterveyslaitoksen Tutkimuksia 4:37–40, 69, 1986 [English summary].
46. Henriks-Eckerman M-L, Laijoki T: Epoksituotteiden sisältämät glysidyylieetterit [Glycidyl ethers in epoxy resin products]. Työterveyslaitoksen Tutkimuksia 4:41–46, 70, 1986 [English summary].
47. Henriksen HR, Petersen HJS: Bedre handsker mod epoxy og andre kemikalier: Beskyttelsesklaeder mod kemikalier [Better gloves against epoxy products and other chemicals: Protective clothing against chemicals]. Copenhagen. Arbejdsmiljöfondet, 1986. [English summary].
48. Herzberg J: Untersuchungen über einen neuen Epoxidkunststoff, "Optyl," zur Herstellung von Brillenfassungen. Berufsdermatosen 21:1–6, 1973.
49. Hine CH, Kodama JK, Anderson HH, et al: The toxicology of epoxy resins. Arch Ind Health 17:129–144, 1958.
50. Hogan DJ, Dannaker CJ, Maibach HI: The prognosis of contact dermatitis. J Am Acad Dermatol 23:300–307, 1990.
51. Holness DL, Nethercott JR: Occupational contact dermatitis due to epoxy resin in a fiberglass binder. J Occup Med 31:87–89, 1989.
52. Holness DL, Nethercott JR: Results of testing with epoxy resin in an occupational health clinic population. Am J Contact Dermatitis 3:169–174, 1992.
53. Ippen H, Mathies V: Die "protrahierte Verätzung" (unter besonderer Berücksichtigung der Hautschäden durch Epoxide und Propansulton). Berufsdermatosen 18:144–165, 1970.
54. Janda R: Synthetic resins. In Gerhartz W, Yamamoto YS, Kaudy L, et al (eds): Ullmann's Encyclopedia of Industrial Chemistry, 5th ed, Vol A8. Weinheim, VCH Verlagsgesellschaft, 1987, pp 277–284.
55. Jolanki R: Occupational skin diseases from epoxy compounds. Epoxy resin compounds, epoxy acrylates and 2,3-epoxypropyl trimethyl ammonium chloride. Acta Derm Venerol 159(Suppl):1–80, 1991.
56. Jolanki R, Estlander T, Henriks-Eckerman M-L, et al: Skin protection and sensitizing epoxy compounds in electron microscopy laboratories. In Mansdorf SZ, Sager R, Nielsen AP (eds): Performance of Protective Clothing: Second Symposium. Philadelphia, American Society for Testing and Materials (ASTM STP 989), 1988, pp 389–395.
57. Jolanki R, Estlander T, Kanerva L: Contact allergy to an epoxy reactive diluent: 1,4-butanediol diglycidyl ether. Contact Dermatitis 16:87–92, 1987.
58. Jolanki R, Estlander T, Kanerva L: Occupational contact dermatitis and contact urticaria caused by epoxy resins. Acta Derm Venerol (Stockh) 134(Suppl):90–94, 1987.
59. Jolanki R, Estlander T, Kanerva L, Tarvainen K: Occupational allergic contact dermatitis caused by a finished reinforced polyester plastic product. In Book of Abstracts, 18th World Congress of Dermatology. New York City, June 12–18, 1992, p 105A.

60. Jolanki R, Kanerva L, Estlander T, Tarvainen K: Concomitact sensitization to triglycidyl isocyanurate, diaminodiphenyl methane and 2-hydroxyethyl methacrylate from silk printing coatings in the manufacture of circuit boards. Contact Dermatitis 1994 (in press).
61. Jolanki R, Kanerva L, Estlander T, et al: Occupational dermatoses from epoxy resin compounds. Contact Dermatitis 23:172–183, 1990.
62. Jolanki R, Sysilampi M-L, Kanerva L, Estlander T: Contact allergy to cycloaliphatic epoxy resins. In Frosch PJ, Dooms-Goossens A, Lachapelle J-M, et al (eds): Current Topics in Contact Dermatitis. Berlin, Springer-Verlag, 1989, pp 360–367.
63. Kanerva L, Estlander T, Jolanki R: Allergic contact dermatitis from dental composite resins due to aromatic epoxy acrylates and aliphatic acrylates. Contact Dermatitis 20:201–211, 1989.
64. Kanerva L, Jolanki R, Estlander T: Allergic contact dermatitis from epoxy resin hardeners. Am J Contact Dermatitis 2:88–97, 1991.
65. Kanerva L, Jolanki R, Estlander T: Allergic contact dermatitis from non-diglycidyl-ether-of-bisphenol-A epoxy resins. Contact Dermatitis 24:293–300, 1991.
66. Kanerva L, Jolanki R, Tupasela O, et al: Immediate and delayed allergy from epoxy resins based on diglycidyl ether of bisphenol A. Scand J Work Environ Health 17:208–215, 1991.
67. Keskinen H: Nordiska expertgruppen för gränsvärdesdokumentation: 92. Organiska syra-anhydrider [Nordic expert group for documentation of occupational exposure limits: 92. Organic acid anhydrides]. Arbete och Hälsa 48:1–33, 1990 [English summary].
68. Kowalska M: Carbon fibre reinforced epoxy prepregs and composites health risks aspects. SAMPE Quarterly 13(2):1–8, 1982.
69. Krajewska D, Rudzki E: Sensitivity to epoxy resins and triethylenetetramine. Contact Dermatitis 2:135–138, 1976.
70. Lichter M, Drury D, Remlinger K: Lichenoid dermatitis caused by epoxy resin. Contact Dermatitis 26:275, 1992.
71. Lynde CW, Warshawski L, Mitchell JC: Screening patch tests in 4190 eczema patients 1972–81. Contact Dermatitis 8:417–421, 1982.
72. Maguire HC: Experimental photoallergic contact dermatitis to bisphenol A. Acta Derm Venerol 68:408–412, 1988.
73. Malanin G, Kalimo K: Facial dermatitis from epoxy resin in a helmet. Contact Dermatitis 12:221, 1985.
74. Malten KE: Tracing back a positive reaction to epoxy resin. Contact Dermatitis 3:217, 1977.
75. Mann RJ, Stewart E, Peachey RDG: Sensitivity to urostomy pouch plastic. Contact Dermatitis 9:80–81, 1983.
76. Mathias CGT: Allergic contact dermatitis from a nonbisphenol A epoxy in a graphite fiber reinforced epoxy laminate. J Occup Med 29:754–755, 1987.
77. Munro CS, Lawrence CM: Occupational contact dermatitis from triglycidyl isocyanurate in a powder paint factory. Contact Dermatitis 26:59, 1992.
78. Muskopf JW, McCollister SB: Epoxy resins. In Gerhartz W, Yamamoto YS, Kaudy L, et al (eds): Ullmann's Encyclopedia of Industrial Chemistry, 5th ed, Vol A9. Weinheim, VCH Verlagsgesellschaft, 1987, pp 547–563.
79. Nakagawa M, Kawai K, Kawai K: Three cases of allergic contact dermatitis from phenylglycidyl-ether. Skin Res 33(Suppl 10):88–95, 1991, [In Japanese with English summary].
80. Nethercott JR: Allergic contact dermatitis due to an epoxy acrylate. Br J Dermatol 104:697–703, 1981.
81. Nishioka K, Ogasawara M, Asagami C: Occupational contact allergy to triglycidyl isocyanurate (TGIC, Tepic^R). Contact Dermatitis 19:379–380, 1988.
82. Peltonen K: Thermal degradation of epoxy powder paints [doctoral dissertation]. Kuopio, Finland, University of Kuopio, 1986.
83. Rebandel P, Rudzki E: Dermatitis caused by epichlorohydrin, oxprenolol hydrochloride and propranolol hydrochloride. Contact Dermatitis 23:199–200, 1990.
84. Richter G, Kadner H: Allergische Kontaktekzeme durch m-Xylylen-diamin in der Polyurethanseidenproduktion. Dermatosen 38:117–120, 1990.
85. Romaguera C, Grimalt F: Pacemaker dermatitis. Contact Dermatitis 7:333, 1981.
86. Rudner EJ: North American group results. Contact Dermatitis 3:208–209, 1977.
87. Rudzki E, Rebandel P: Dermatitis from methyl 2,3 epoxy-3-(4-methoxyphenyl)propionate. Contact Dermatitis 23:382, 1990.
88. Rycroft RJG: Atypical psoriasis following epoxy resin sensitization. J Soc Occup Med 30:132–134, 1980.
89. Savla M: Epoxy resin adhesives. In Skeist I (ed): Handbook of Adhesives, 2nd ed. New York, Van Nostrand Reinhold, 1977, pp 434–464.

90. Senff H, Kuhlwein A, Hausen BM: Allergisches Kontaktekzem auf Dicyandiamid. Dermatosen 36:99–101, 1988.
91. Srinivas CR, Devadiga R, Aroor AR: Footwear dermatitis due to bisphenol A. Contact Dermatitis 20:150–151, 1989.
92. Storrs FJ, Rosenthal LE, Adams RM, et al: Prevalence and relevance of allergic reactions in patients patch tested in North America—1984 to 1985. J Am Acad Dermatol 20:1038–1045, 1989.
93. Suhonen R: Epoxy-dermatitis in a ski-stick factory. Contact Dermatitis 9:131–133, 1983.
94. Tarvainen K, Jolanki R, Forsman-Grönholm L, et al: Exposure, skin protection and occupational skin diseases in the glass fibre reinforced plastics industry. Contact Dermatitis 29:119–127, 1993.
95. Thorgeirsson A: Sensitization capacity of epoxy reactive diluents in the guinea pig. Acta Derm Venerol 58:329–331, 1978.
96. Thorgeirsson A: Sensitization capacity of epoxy resin hardeners in the guinea pig. Acta Derma Venerol 58:332–336, 1978.
97. Thorgeirsson A, Fregert S: Allergenicity of epoxy resins in the guinea pig. Acta Derm Venerol 57:253–256, 1977.
98. Thorgeirsson A, Fregert S, Ramnäs O: Sensitization capacity of epoxy resin oligomers in the guinea pig. Acta Derm Venerol 58:17–21, 1978.
99. Toome BK: Allergic contact dermatitis to a nasal cannula. Arch Dermatol 125:571, 1989.
100. Tosti A, Guerra L, Bardazzi F: Occupational contact dermatitis from exposure to epoxy resins and acrylates. Clin Dermatol 10:133–140, 1992.
101. Vanherle G, Smith DC (eds): Posterior Composite Resin Dental Restorative Materials. St. Paul, Minnesota Mining and Manufacturing Co., 1985.
102. Van Joost T, Roesyanto ID, Satyawan I: Occupational sensitization to epichlorohydrin (ECH) and bisphenol-A during the manufacture of epoxy resin. Contact Dermatitis 22:125–126, 1990.
103. Wilkinson DS, Budden MG, Hambly EM: A 10-year review of an industrial dermatitis clinic. Contact Dermatitis 6:11–17, 1980.
104. Woytoń A, Wasik F, Blizanowska A: Niezwykla reakcja anafilaktyczna i wypryskowa po kontakcie z zywicami epoksydowymi [An uncommon anaphylactic and eczematous reaction after contact with epoxide resins]. Przegl Dermatol 61:303–308, 1974.

JACK N. MOSS

RECONCILING CLINICAL DATA WITH RISK: THE KATHON® BIOCIDE STORY

Product stewardship in today's culture encompasses a quality management strategy of inordinate complexity to ensure product integrity from the point of production through end-use application and ultimate entry into the environment as a waste product.

Inherent in a total product stewardship program is the identification of risks, real as well as perceived, associated with the product prior to its introduction into the marketplace (Table 1). Once the needs are anticipated, the hazards are identified, the risks are characterized, and a determination of the acceptability of such risks is defined, the risk management process is subsequently triggered. Within this framework, the central focus of the program is on product safety, since a sound and effective program in product safety not only minimizes real risk but also makes good business sense. Thus, any program that carefully and methodically characterizes and successfully manages risks associated with new products must be an ambitious one. This chapter discusses the approach employed by Rohm and Haas Co. to shepherd an extremely effective microbicide through the stages of risk analysis and management, with special emphasis on the role played by clinical evaluation. The risk analysis process for a microbicide with broad applications as well as varied human exposure patterns involves planning stages similar to those associated with the development of new drugs.

Before the chapter details the specifics of the program described herein, it is important to review the foundation of the product safety

OCCUPATIONAL MEDICINE: State of the Art Reviews—
Vol. 9, No. 1, January–March 1994. Philadelphia, Hanley & Belfus, Inc.

TABLE 1. Elements of Product Stewardship

• Anticipation
• Hazard identification
• Risk analysis/risk assessment
• Risk management

program and note that the elements of a risk analysis/risk management program are not necessarily unique to Rohm and Haas Co. Many, if not most, major chemical corporations have adopted similar techniques to ensure product integrity and safety. The concept is not new; health risk assessments were formally introduced by the U.S. Food and Drug Administration in 1972 as part of the overall regulatory process for new drugs. Similarly, in 1976 the U.S. Environmental Protection Agency (EPA) became the first agency to promulgate guidelines for the scientific assessment of cancer risks associated with new as well as established chemicals.

Risk is defined as the likelihood of the occurrence of an adverse event and its consequences on human health or the environment.

The early determinants of chemical risk to human health are functions of the likely exposure and the intrinsic toxicological properties of the chemical as determined by controlled, nonclinical toxicity tests.

Table 2, taken from the EPA and National Academy of Science lists the major components of the risk assessment process to ensure the prudent use of any chemical and its safety in commerce. The risk assessment process relies predominantly, but not exclusively, on those components. An unassessed or underassessed risk characterization of any chemical carries a high level of potential risk to human health.

Early in the Rohm and Haas Co. biocide research program it was observed that a candidate compound from a chemical class of isothiazolones exhibited extraordinary broad-spectrum antimicrobial activity in vitro against bacteria, fungi, and algae. Low inhibitory concentrations ranging from 1 to 10 ppm, to achieve effective microbial control, positioned this compound as a likely preservative for a variety of broad-based applications. Stability coupled with efficacy allowed for its consideration in industrial systems such as metalworking coolants, as well as in consumer applications such as cosmetics and toiletries. The structure of the candidate isothiazolone is shown below. It is a 75:25% by weight mixture of 5-chloro-2-methyl-4-isothiazolin-3-one and 2-methyl-4-isothiazolin-3-one, herein designated as "MCI/MI."

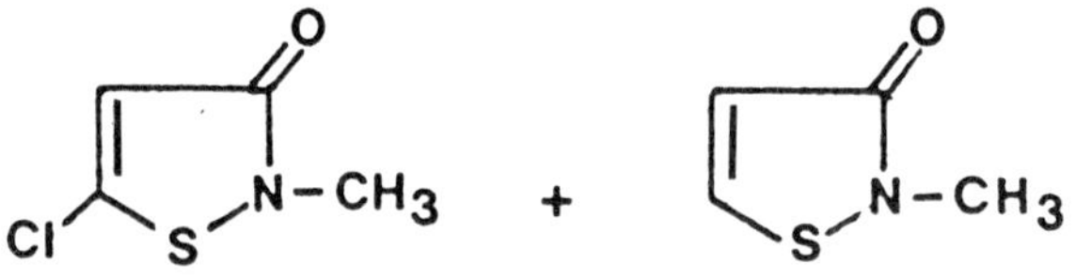

MCI + MI

Thus an extensive nonclinical toxicological assessment was launched in accordance with those requirements for internal risk assessment as well as for chemical registration. The details of each study are not the subject of this review;

TABLE 2. Major Components of Risk Assessment Process

Hazard assessment	—	Nonclinical data
Dose responses	—	Relationships between dose and reactions
Exposure assessment	—	Likelihood and frequency
Risk characterization	—	Adverse health effects vs. exposure scenarios

however, the major studies required for hazard evaluations are summarized in Table 3.

A review of the nonclinical data resulted in the conclusion that the principal "intrinsic" hazard or risk associated with exposure to this compound was a concentration-dependent irritant effect on exposed tissue, with high concentrations resulting in "chemical burns." Subsequent special testing for sensitization potential also revealed that MCI/MI produced delayed contact hypersensitivity in animal models. The Buehler guinea pig test was employed as the primary test because, like the repeat-insult patch test, it is predictive for human contact sensitization potential. Since delayed contact hypersensitivity is a cell-mediated immunological process associated with interactions of haptenic materials, skin macrophages, and T lymphocytes, the mouse lymph node cell proliferation assay was also used to assess sensitization potential. Most contact allergens stimulate lymph node T-cell proliferation in a concentration-dependent manner, as indicated by an increase in (^{3}H) methyl thymidine incorporated into DNA. MCI/MI in this test system also induced T-cell proliferation, confirming its potential to act as a classical contact allergen.

Traditionally, these nonclinical tests may be useful in predicting sensitization potential and relative sensitization potency; thus they are valuable models for hazard classification. However, their use in extrapolating to man for risk assessment purposes is limited because they maximize concentration and exposure and fail to address the complexity and array of human exposure, vehicle dependency, partitioning, and so on. It is within this frame of reference that predictive testing in human subjects becomes a primary consideration as a tool to assess as well as to minimize consumer risk. Since the sentinel human health hazard of MCI/MI exposure appeared to be associated with its cutaneous and mucous membrane effects, the focus of the product stewardship program was directed to both qualitative and quantitative assessment of these risks.

The importance of contact dermatitis is emphasized by the number of reports in which skin problems account for a significant portion of all occupational diseases. Allergic contact dermatitis probably accounts for about 25% of the occupational cases studied. Although not a life-threatening condition, it has been recognized as an important risk factor in certain occupations.

TABLE 3. Nonclinical Toxicological Profile of MCI/MI

- Acute through chronic toxicity
- Biochemical transformation
- Genotoxicity
- Teratogenesis
- Carcinogenesis
- Sensitization potential

Despite their frequent use and ubiquitousness, cosmetics and toiletries probably account for a surprisingly small percentage of the cases of allergic contact dermatitis seen in clinics, with fragrances and preservatives probably accounting for one-half of the cases. This suggests that most products can be formulated with potential sensitizers at levels that are effective in achieving their end-use application at concentrations below sensitization thresholds.

Like most biological effects, cell-mediated contact allergy is a dose-related phenomenon highly dependent on the dose density at the contact site. Evidence for this dependency was shown in human volunteer studies with dinitrochlorobenzene in which induction as well as elicitation was a function of the dose of hapten. Similarly, a threshold for elicitation was also demonstrated for individuals previously shown to be sensitized to formaldehyde. These findings were consistent with earlier animal studies with MCI/MI in which a zone of nonresponsiveness was suggested by the data on induction and elicitation concentrations. Thus, despite their sensitizing capacity, these observations on dose-related responsiveness and the likelihood that there are concentrations below which sensitization does not occur suggested their use even in high-pattern-exposure scenarios such as cosmetics and toiletries.

Animal models such as the Buehler guinea pig sensitization test and the relatively new mouse local lymph node assay are invaluable tools for measurement of intrinsic sensitization potential as well as relative sensitization potency. However, the ultimate assessment of sensitization risk for the worker and consumer is best made through the use of controlled, clinical safety studies in human volunteers to assess the irritation and sensitization thresholds of candidate products. Evidence for the need for clinical assessment has been demonstrated by the observation that methylene bis thiocyanate is an apparent "strong" sensitizer in guinea pigs but that sensitization in humans is rare. Similarly, nickel, a common cause of contact allergy in humans, is difficult to detect in animal models.

A qualitative exposure assessment was next undertaken, since the end use of this biocide covered an array of commercial and consumer applications. Table 4 summarizes these exposure patterns. It was obvious just from this short list of potential exposures that the patterns were varied and ubiquitous, with worst-case or high-exposure patterns, represented by such applications as coolant systems and leave-on cosmetic and toiletry products. It is not uncommon for metalworkers to have their hands exposed to coolant several hours per day during their workweek. Similarly, high-exposure patterns are common with cosmetic and toiletry products when large and diversified populations may be exposed to many products daily for long periods of time. Thus, the risk associated with such exposures was subsequently assessed through clinical evaluations of irritation and sensitization under controlled and exaggerated-exposure conditions relative to worker or consumer exposure.

TABLE 4. Skin-Exposure Patterns Relative to Use

High	Medium	Low
Metalworking coolants	Paint	Cooling tower water
Spray cleaners	Textiles	Paper mill pulps
Swimming pools	Oil fields	Fuels
Leave-on cosmetics	Dishwashing liquids	Rinse-off cosmetics/toiletries

Predictive tests for early assessment of irritancy thresholds and for sensitization potential made use of occlusive patch testing in normal human volunteers free of obvious skin disease. Protocols for such studies were based on classical 21-day cumulative irritancy tests and the Draize assay, which provides for the application of MCI/MI in various vehicles under exaggerated conditions of exposure. Not only does such predictive testing allow for an early assessment of risk, but it also provides two other important elements in the risk characterization process: (1) it allows for calculation of an arbitrary safety factor to be applied for end use of the chemical, and (2) it allows for selection of an optimal concentration of the biocide for use in diagnostic testing.

Results from human cumulative irritancy and Draize testing on MCI/MI suggested threshold concentrations in the range of 100–200 ppm of active ingredient in either an aqueous or a petrolatum vehicle. Effective-use concentrations of the biocide in the majority of either industrial or consumer products ranged from 3 to 15 ppm of active ingredient, with an average of about 10 ppm (Table 5).

Although a safety factor of 10 may be acceptable for certain biocides with potential sensitization risks, ultimate acceptability of such risk is best determined through product safety testing. Such trials are normally conducted by prudent formulators by means of repeat-insult patch tests of products containing the biocide at use concentrations or through use tests under controlled and sometimes exaggerated-use conditions. These studies provide a benchmark for establishing sensitization risk in the normal population and help to define the dose-response relationship associated with the use of the biocide. However, the likelihood and frequency of contact allergies surfacing in the population following long periods of either indirect or purposeful exposure may not be fully answered through short-term-exposure studies or by extrapolation from low-dose-exposure models. The need for such information triggered the risk management process, with special emphasis on surveillance (Table 6).

Risk management as it applied to the management of this biocide with its proclivity to induce allergic contact dermatitis involves not only the mandates of the regulatory process but also the manufacturer's awareness of the socioeconomic impact of the chemical so that decisions can be made on selective as well as general use of the product.

The decision-making process became markedly enhanced by introduction of the surveillance initiative in the overall product stewardship program. While hazard communication and exposure reduction, particularly in the workplace, was adequately handled by means of technical brochures, workplace seminars, and video programs, the surveillance program afforded the opportunity for continuous risk analysis with the result that exposure scenarios, as well as end uses, could be modified in a timely fashion, thus minimizing risks to the chemical. The surveillance initiative had three objectives: (1) to ensure that the recommended-use levels were adhered to in the final product, (2) to monitor complaint rates, and (3) to assess the prevalence rates of sensitization in clinical populations.

TABLE 5. Arbitrary Safety Factor for MCI/MI

Highest nonirritating/ nonsensitizing concentration	= 100 ppm
Effective-use concentration	= 3–15 ppm (x = 10 ppm)
Safety factor	= ~10

TABLE 6. Elements of Risk Management

• Hazard communication
• Hazard reduction
• Exposure reduction
• Surveillance

The first objective was met by the establishment of service laboratories in key regions, such as the United States, Europe, and Japan, to provide analytical expertise for end users and to ensure that end-use concentrations were within recommended limits. The misting of cutting oils into the metalworking atmosphere is a normal occurrence; thus air monitoring was another segment of the surveillance program.

For consumer products such as toiletries, excursions from the recommended-use levels were sometimes noted. Random selection of products from the shelf for analysis allowed subsequent alerts to the formulators to modify their products accordingly.

Complaint-rate monitoring, particularly in the workplace setting, is an ongoing process handled through corporate health and safety groups and focused particularly on accidental exposure attributed to spills, mishandling, or misuse.

The third objective of the surveillance program was the measurement of sensitization prevalence rates. This provided a direct means by which contact allergy to this preservative could be detected in the clinical population. Further, the approach allows separation of the perceived from the real risk by considering prevalence sensitization rates in clinical populations as a function of time and the amount of biocide in commerce. This program was initiated by means of a cooperative effort with dermatologists specializing in contact allergy in a clinical setting, who use diagnostic patch testing as a routine procedure in their clinical practice.

Despite imperfections, the assessment of sensitization prevalence rates in clinical populations by means of diagnostic patch testing continues to be a useful gauge of product safety when allergic contact dermatitis is the principal health effect. With refinements in experimental design, diagnostic patch testing is especially useful in tracking product safety over time. Four such studies were conducted with MCI/MI: two in the United States, one in Europe, and one in Japan by means of a cooperative effort with leading patch test clinics in each region. An earlier multicenter study in the United States was conducted independently by the North American Contact Dermatitis Group.

Each of these studies was designed to compare prevalence rates concomitantly with other preservative systems in commerce, since multiple allergies are not an uncommon finding. In order to help establish the relevance of each patch-positive response, titrations of the biocide were conducted in these patients, and, when feasible, relevance was also assessed by means of double-blind provocative-use testing with generic products with and without the biocide. Skin sensitivity was assessed by the clinician in accordance with standard arbitrary grading scores.

Despite clinic-to-clinic variation, there emerged a clear picture of sensitization rates in the clinical population, thus demonstrating that the prevalence rate for sensitization attributed to MCI/MI had stabilized at levels no higher, and most times lower, than most preservatives in commerce today. The significance of the surveillance program is probably best illustrated by a comparison of the relationship between the current prevalence rate of sensitization to MCI/MI and the total amount of biocide in commerce in the United States. Despite significant increases in the amount of biocide sold for industrial and consumer use, no changes in sensitization rates have been observed over a seven- to eight-year monitoring period.

As previously noted, allergic contact dermatitis accounts for about 25% of occupation-related contact dermatitis, whereas allergy to cosmetics and toiletries is thought to be responsible for about 5% of the allergies seen in clinics. It is therefore incumbent upon prudent and responsible manufacturers of chemicals to adopt a product stewardship program that allows for early detection of potential health hazards, both characterizing the potential risks and, subsequently, managing them in a way that reduces or minimizes any further increase in sensitization risk.

The program described herein adheres to those principles of product stewardship that facilitate the development and implementation of appropriate actions to monitor and reduce risk levels. The ultimate success of the program was achieved through the cooperative efforts of the dermatology community's working hand in hand with industry.

REFERENCES

1. Adams RM: Occupational Skin Disease, 2nd ed. Philadelphia, W.B. Saunders, 1990.
2. Adams RM: Patch testing: A recapitulation. J Am Acad Dermatol 5:629–643, 1981.
3. Adams RM, et al: A five-year study of cosmetic reactions. J Am Acad Dermatol 13:1062–1069, 1985.
4. Basketter DA, et al: Structure-activity relationship in contact allergy. Int J Cosm Sci 12:81, 1990.
5. Buehler EV: Delayed contact hypersensitivity in the guinea pig. Arch Dermatol 91:171, 1965.
6. Buell D: Industry's perspective on how risk management is working. In Risk Management of Existing Chemicals. Washington, DC, CMA Seminar, 1983.
7. Chan PK: Kathon biocide: Manifestation of delayed contact dermatitis in guinea pigs is dependent on the concentration for induction and challenge. J Invest Dermatol 81:409–411, 1983.
8. Curtis GL: Clinical safety testing of cosmetics and personal care products. J Toxicol Cutan Ocul Toxicol 10:279–287, 1991.
9. Deisler PF Jr: Risk assessment: Introduction and overview in risk analysis in the chemical industry. Washington, DC, CMA Seminar, 1985.
10. Gad SC: A scheme for prediction and ranking of relative potencies of dermal sensitizers. J Appl Toxicol 8:361–368, 1988.
11. Jayjock MA, et al: Low-applied-dose extrapolation of induction and elicitation of contact allergy. Am J Contemp Dermatol 3:86–91, 1982.
12. Kimber I, et al: The local lymph node assay. Fd Chem Toxicol 30:165–169, 1992.
13. Marks JG Jr: MCI/MI (Kathon CG biocide)—U.S. multicenter study of human skin sensitization. Am J Contemp Dermatol 1:157–161, 1990.
14. Marks JG Jr, et al: Contact and Occupational Dermatology. St. Louis, Mosby/Year Book, 1992.
15. Marks JG Jr, et al: MCI/MI—Second U.S. multicenter study of human skin sensitization. In press.
16. Menne T, et al: Contact sensitization to 5-chloro-2-methyl-4 isothiazolin-3-one and 2-methyl-4-isothiazolin-3-one (MCI/MI). Contact Dermatitis 24:334–341, 1991.
17. Munro IC, et al: Risk assessment and regulatory decision making. Fd Cosmet Toxicol 19:549–560, 1981.
18. Neal SB: Int Biodeter 26:259–271, 1990.
19. Press F: Risk Assessment in the Federal Government: Managing the Process. Washington, DC, National Academy Press, 1983.
20. Rietschel RL, et al: MCI/MI reactions in patients screened for vehicle and preservative hypersensitivity. J Am Acad Dermatol 22:734–738, 1990.
21. Robinson MK, et al: A risk assessment process for allergic contact sensitization. Fd Chem Toxicol 27:479–489, 1989.
22. Rodericks JV: In Proceedings of the Risk Assessment Symposium, CTFA Series, 1, 1982.
23. Shuster S: Patch-test sensitivity and reproducibility in individuals and populations. Am J Contemp Dermatol 3:74–78, 1992.

INDEX

Entries in **boldface type** indicate complete articles.